HEALTH, ILLNESS AND HEALING

THEMES AND ISSUES IN MEDICAL ANTHROPOLOGY

HEALTH, ILLNESS AND HEALING

THEMES AND ISSUES IN MEDICAL ANTHROPOLOGY

K.E. RAJ PRAMUKH

SERIALS PUBLICATIONS
NEW DELHI (INDIA)

First Published – 2009

ISBN: 978-81-8387-184-6

Published by

SERIALS PUBLICATIONS
4830/24, Prahlad Street, Ansari Road
Darya Ganj, New Delhi-110002 (India)
Phone : 23245225 Fax : 91-11-23272135
E-mail: serials@satyam.net.in

CONTENTS

PREFACE

This book is designed to deal with the critical themes and issues in Medical Anthropology. Medical Anthropology is an interdisciplinary bio-cultural discipline cutting across the boundaries of Epidemiology, Sociology, Human Genetics and Community Medicine including Public Health.

Anthropological orientations in studying human behaviour related to health and illness offer useful insights to physicians, researchers and paramedical staff working especially in remote tribal and rural areas. Anthropological sophistication fosters a questioning attitude towards medical practices, modern as well as traditional, which may be introduced in the un/under developed areas where the natives culture is taken for granted by the planners without adequate support from well controlled studies.

Although this book is intended to be a source book for all the researchers and teachers of Anthropology in Indian Universities and Colleges at various levels, all those who are working in the area of health, illness and healing, it is hoped, would find it useful in some way or other. The last chapter on paradigms of health and the contexts of marginalization without doubt would be of interest to many others.

Some of the chapters in this book were published earlier in journals of repute. A few new chapters were added to make reading a meaningful continuity without loosing the focus. The account on AIDS was taken from Graham Pembrey's note on the internet based on an original article by Jenni Fredriksson-Bass and Annabel Kanabus. My grateful thanks to him.

Many of my Research Scholars have helped me in different capacities at various points of time. I would like to express my appreciation particularly for a few of them namely: Mr.K.Sanyasi Naidu, Miss.I.Jhansi Rani, Mrs.R.Ramanamma and Mr.D.V.S.S.Appala Naidu. I am also thankful to Mr. V.Devanand for his assistance related to computer editing and also to Mr.N.Elisha for his typing services. Finally, I only hope that my students would be immensely benefited by this work among others.

K.E. Raj Pramukh

INTRODUCTION

Health is a subject of study for many disciplines including Anthropology. Medical Anthropology studies health which is a relatively new branch of Anthropology with a bio-cultural perspective integrating both medical science and biology with the social and behavioral sciences. It deals with the explanations of the causes of ill health people believe in different cultures, the specialists from whom they receive the treatment and the type of treatment for different illnesses. It constructs illness in terms of the culture of the people it studies. It also studies these beliefs and practices as they are related to the psychological and bio-social dimensions of the human organism in relation to health and disease.

For a better and comprehensive understanding of the subject, it is necessary to know something about the discipline of Anthropology itself, of which Medical Anthropology is a branch. The term, 'Anthropology' is derived from the Greek, meaning 'the study of man-human beings'. Anthropology is considered as the 'most scientific of the humanities and the most humane of the sciences'. Gerald Weiss (1973:1381) defined Anthropology as, "the study of sum total of all human phenomena, everywhere across the face of the planet and beyond, and through all time....". Anthropology has been referred to as (1) a 'natural or biological science' in that it studies the physical evolution and biological nature of human beings; (2) a 'social science', in that it studies the behaviour of human beings as members of social groups; (3) a 'historical' discipline, in that it seeks to reconstruct sequences in cultural development; and (4) one of the 'humanities', in that it studies art, folklore, oral tradition and so on. Holism, comparativism and relativism are the fundamental orientations of Anthropological studies. As a holistic study, Anthropology encompasses every aspect of human beings. Thus, while other disciplines are interested in studying a particular aspect of human beings, Anthropology brings into its scope all biological and socio-cultural aspects concerning human beings: their origins, development, social and political organizations, religions, languages, art and artifacts, etc., Social Anthropology has been called as comparative sociology by Radcliffe-Brown emphasizing the fact that it indulges in cross-cultural comparisons of different varieties of cultures. 'Relativism', makes Anthropological studies shun from making value judgements while studying the native cultures. Every culture is studied in the context of that particular culture only treating all cultures on par.

Anthropology, as an academic discipline, has several branches. Franz Boas introduced the four-fold division of Anthropology in American Universities. His wide interests, spanning from biological anthropology to linguistics gave American anthropology a topical breadth which is not present in Great Britain or France, where Anthropology is pre-eminently Social Anthropology, where as Archaeology and Biological Anthropology are separate fields.

Franz Boas's four-fold division includes Cultural Anthropology, Physical Anthropology, Prehistoric Anthropology and Linguistic Anthropology. Accordingly, Physical Anthropology–also known as human biology or biological Anthropology–is the study of the evolution of the human species, and is concerned with explaining the causes for the present diversity of human populations. Prehistoric Anthropology utilizes the techniques of archaeology, paleontology, genetics and serology, as well as the study of primate behaviour and ecology. Cultural Anthropology deals with the ideational aspects including the material culture, which include the art and artifacts of mankind, both in the present and the past. It includes studies of the arts, musical instruments, weapons, clothes, tools and agricultural implements of different populations, and all other aspects of the technology that human beings use to control, shape, exploit and enhance their social or natural environments. Cultural Anthropology also deals with the comparative study of present-day human societies and their cultural systems. Linguistic Anthropology deals with the structure of language and the structure of societies by providing a source of ideas and models that might have value in the descriptions and analysis of culture. It is held that cultural classifications of reality are built up and organized in the same way as language. The culture of a people is related to their language. Some aspects of language, particularly lexicon, reflect the cultural importance of subjects, people, objects, and natural phenomena. Some Anthropologists have argued that the language a people speak predisposes them to see the world in a certain way by shaping their perceptions of reality. This idea known as 'Sapir-Whorf' hypothesis argues that the lexicon of a language influences perceptions by leading its speakers to filter out a certain objective properties of reality in favour of other properties. Linguistic Anthropology also is the study of how speech is influenced by cultural factors, including culturally defined contexts and situations, the goals of the speaker, the presence of other parties and so forth.

Social Anthropology is the dominant approach in the United Kingdom emphasizing the social dimensions of human life. Man is a social animal, organized into groups that regulate and perpetuate themselves, and it is man's experience as a member of society that shapes his view of the world. In this perspective culture is seen as one of the important ways that man organizes and legitimizes his society, and provides the basis for its social, political and economic organization. In the USA, cultural anthropology focuses more on the systems of symbols, ideas and meanings that comprise a culture, and of which social organization is just an expression. In practice, the differences in emphasis of social and cultural anthropology provide valuable and complementary perspectives on two central issues–the ways that human groups organize themselves, and the ways that they view the world they inhabit. In other words, when studying a group of human beings it is necessary to study the features of both their society and their culture (Helman, 2001:1).

'Keesing (1981:518) has defined a society as 'a population marked by relative separation from surrounding populations and a distinctive culture'. The boundaries between societies are sometimes vague, but in general each has its own territorial and political identity. In studying any society, Anthropologists investigate how the members of that society organize themselves into different groups, hierarchies and roles. The underlying rules of the organization of a society and the ways that it is symbolized and transmitted are all part of that society's *culture.*

The Concept of Culture

Culture is the key concept in Anthropology and more than 250 (Kroeber and Kluckhohn, 1963) definitions have been given by different Anthropologists. Perhaps the most famous and the earliest being Tylor's definition in his 'Primitive Culture' (1871): 'Culture or civilization, taken in its wide ethnographic sense, is that complex whole which includes knowledge, belief, art, morals, law, custom and any other capabilities and habits acquired by man as a member of society'.

An important point in understanding the role of culture is that it must always be seen in its particular context. This context is made up of historical, economic, social, political and geographical factors, and means that the culture of any group of people, at any particular point in time, is always influenced by many other factors.

For example, economic factors are an important cause of ill health, since poverty may result in poor nutrition, overcrowded living conditions, inadequate clothing, physical and psychological violence, psychological stress, and drug and alcohol abuse. The unequal distribution of economic resources, both between countries and within each country itself, can lead to this situation. In the developing countries too, whatever the local culture, poor health is usually associated with a low income, since this influences the sort of food, water, clothing, sanitation, housing and medical care that people are able to afford. For example, Unterhalter's (1982:617-36) study of infant mortality rates among different ethnic communities in

Johannesburg, South Africa, between 1910 and 1979 found very much higher rates among blacks and other non-white groups than among whites, and this clearly correlated with the economic and social inequalities imposed on them by the apartheid system. Preston-Whyte (1995:315-37) has described how the legacy of this political system has made the control of AIDS in South Africa much more difficult today. This is because apartheid system in the rural areas, often separated men from their wives, sending them to work in the cities for many years. Here they lived in male-only hostels, and this helped institutionalize multiple- partner sex relationships for many of them. At the same time, back in the rural areas poor women sometimes had to depend on selling sex to earn money for their own survival and that of their children. Therefore, culture should never be considered in a vacuum, but only as one component of a complex mix of influences on what people believe and how they live their lives. A final misuse of the concept of culture–especially in medical care–is that its influence may be over-emphasized in interpreting how some people present their symptoms to health professionals. Symptoms or behaviour may be ascribed to the person's culture, when they are not really due to an underlying physical or mental disorder. Similarly, physical disorders may be confused with mental illness in certain cultural contexts. Thus Weis (1985:121-200) has described how, in India and elsewhere, some cases of cerebral malaria have been mistakenly diagnosed as mental illness.

Medical Anthropology

Although Medical Anthropology is a branch of Social and Cultural Anthropology its roots also could be found deep within Medicine and other natural sciences, for it is concerned with a wide range of biological phenomena, especially in relation to health and disease. As a subject it lies sometimes uncomfortably–in the overlap between the social and natural sciences, and draws its insights from both sets of disciplines.

Anthropologists studying the socio-cultural factors have pointed out that, in all human societies, beliefs and practices relating to ill health are a central feature of the culture. Often these are linked to beliefs about the origin of a much wider range of misfortunes (including accidents, interpersonal conflicts, natural disasters, crop failures, theft and loss), of which ill health is just one form. In some societies the whole range of these misfortunes is blamed on supernatural forces, or on divine retribution, or on the malevolence of a witch or sorcerer. The values and customs associated with ill health are part of the wider culture, and cannot really be studied in isolation from it. One cannot really understand how people react to illness, death or other misfortunes without an understanding of the type of culture they have grown up in or acquired. In addition to the study of culture it is also necessary to examine the organization of health and illness in that society (the health care system), which includes the ways in which people have become recognized as ill, the ways that they present this illness to other people, the attributes of those they present their illness to, and the ways that the illness is dealt with. This group of 'healers' is found in different forms in every human society. Anthropologists are particularly interested in the characteristics of this special social group; their selection, training, concepts, values and internal organization. They also study the way these people fit into the social system as a whole–their rank in the social hierarchy, their economic or political power, and the division of labour between them and other members of the society. In some societies the healers play roles beyond their healing functions also acting as 'integrators' of the society, who regularly reassert the society's values or as agents of social control, helping to label and punish socially deviant behaviour. Their focus may not be only on the ill individual, but rather on his 'ill' family, community, village or tribe. It is therefore important when studying how individuals in a particular society perceive and react to ill health, and the types of health care that they turn to, to know something about both the cultural and the social attributes of the society in which they live. This is one of the main tasks of Medical Anthropology. Chapter VII of this book gives a vivid description of the Shaman and the divine healers.

At the biological end of the spectrum, Medical Anthropology draws on the techniques and findings of Medical science and its various sub-fields such as microbiology, biochemistry, genetics, parasitology, pathology, nutrition and epidemiology. It is possible to link biological changes found by these techniques to social and cultural factors in a particular society. For example, a hereditary disease transmitted by a recessive gene may occur at a higher frequency in a particular population due to that group's cultural preference for endogamy, that is, for marrying only within one's own family or local kin group. To understand these problems, one needs the following perspectives (Helman 2001:5): Clinical medicine (to identify the clinical manifestation of the disease), pathology (to confirm the disease on the cellular or biochemical level), genetics (to identify and predict the hereditary basis of the disease and its linkage to a recessive gene), epidemiology (to show its high incidence in a particular population in relation to 'pooling' of recessive genes and certain marriage customs), and social or cultural Anthropology (to explain the marriage patterns of that society and to identify who may marry whom within it).

Helman (2001:1-11) gives an excellent account of the scope of Medical Anthropology emphasizing the important role of cultural factors in Health and Disease. He portrayed the study of human life cycle as an area of research interest to medical anthropologists, specifically mentioning childhood and old age. Von Mering and Kasdan (1970) edited a book in which the chapters represent summary statements emphasizing how anthropology relates to the health sciences. Medical Anthropology, thus, utilizes the findings of social-cultural anthropology and biological sciences as well by being a 'bio-cultural' discipline.

1

ANTHROPOLOGY AND HEALTH

Anthropology is described as a 'holistic' discipline, which emphasizes the total social and cultural context in the explanation of the behaviour of human groups. The World Health Organization's (WHO) definition of health reflects this very concept of 'holism'. Accordingly, in 1948 WHO defined health as, 'a state of complete physical, mental and social well being of an individual and it is not merely the absence of disease or infirmity'.

Foster and Anderson (1978:2-3) defined Medical Anthropology as: 'A bio-cultural discipline concerned with both the biological and socio-cultural aspects of human behavior, and particularly with the ways in which the two interacted throughout human history to influence health and disease'. The bio-cultural nature of medical Anthropology is evident in a number of review articles (Caudill, 1953; Polgar, 1962; Fabrega Jr,1972; Colson and Selby, 1974; Landy(ed), 1980).

Fabrega, Jr, (1972:2-3) emphasizing the role of cultural factor defined it, as 'a medical anthropological inquiry is that (a) elucidates the factors, mechanisms, and processes that play a role in or influence the way in which individuals and groups are affected by and respond to illness and disease, and (b) examines these problems with an emphasis on patterns of behaviour'. Primary emphasis is given to studies that are conducted in non-western settings and that rely on the concept of culture.

Anthropological researches around the world have generated a rich body of knowledge concerning health and disease resulting in the delineation of areas critical for our study and further probe. As a first step, differentiating the terms 'disease' and 'illness' from each other has been made, as 'science' demands precision in the universal standardization of the terms. Disease, accordingly, refers to pathological states of the organism, whether or not they are culturally or psychologically recognized, where as Illness refers to culturally or socially defined or conditioned perceptions and experiences of ill health, including some states which may be defined as diseases and others which are not classifiable in terms of medical definitions of pathological states. Accordingly, disease is now universally referred to as a western bio-medical term while illness is culturally defined and identified with the local indigenous knowledge (Fabrega,Jr, 1972:167). Sickness is a general global term, which refers to all events involving ill health. This differentiation is made possible by the rich body of indigenous knowledge generated by the countless field endeavors carried out by innumerable Anthropologists all around the world, mostly among the isolated, un/under developed, illiterate, tribal/rural communities since the turn of the twentieth century. Eventually, a new branch of Anthropology, 'Medical Anthropology', emerged and by the beginning of 1980s it is offered as a specialization in many western and non-western Universities as well.

Anthropology and Medicine

A medical system exists as a part of a larger network of socio-cultural system. According to Parsons (1951) a medical system as a social system should have the four functional imperatives viz., adaptation, goal-orientation, integration and latency. As a cultural system one has to analyze the beliefs, values and attitudes, which are functionally related to sickness and death. Medical Anthropology unravels the dynamics of illness, sickness, disease and health in the total context of social structure. Although biological implications of medicine are too evident, the fact that medical systems interact with social factors cannot be ignored. Precisely for this reason the great German scholar Virchow during the 1840s described medicine as a social science.

As Anthropology studies small scale societies like the tribals, two dimensions could be easily found in the Anthropological approaches to study the tribal medicine: to consider tribal medicine, as (1) a cultural complex, of material objects, tools, techniques, ideas and values, and as (2) a part of social structure and organization, i.e., the network of relations between groups, classes and categories. It is now increasingly realized that a knowledge of these two aspects of medicine, in itself and in relation to other aspects of social life such as political economy, religion, magic and law is necessary to understand the culture of any society. These approaches also help us to understand the social dynamics as to why certain elements of modern medicine are easily accepted and why others are rejected.

The social dynamics approach has facilitated some scholars to study the indigenous medical practices epistemologically. Khare (1963), for example, studied the indigenous medical practices in the framework of 'parochialization' and 'sanskritization' demonstrating how the upper castes try to relate their etiology in terms of great tradition where as the lower castes define them in terms of lesser gods and deities. There were also a few studies which were very critical about the functioning of medical establishments. The 'Theory of Gaze' formulated by Foucault (1975) is one of the most radical theoretical formulations in which he traces historically how the medical system in the west has operated in the feudal capitalist environment and eventually made the medical profession as an industry–by dehumanizing it. More often than not, the physicians tended to reduce the patient as a specimen of laboratory experimentation. Ivan Illich's 'Medical Nemesis' (1974) is another powerful critique of the medical establishments. Illich challenged the fundamental premise of medical 'progress', arguing that institutional medicine is overwhelmingly pathogenic and actively 'sickening'. David Wootton (2006) takes an unsparing interest in why doctors made bad decisions, ignored seemingly obvious discoveries and consistently refused to adopt therapies that stood to be of the greatest benefit to mankind. " We can only think about medical progress if we start with the long tradition of medical failure ... we know how to write histories of stasis, of delay, of digression". His book 'Bad medicine: Doctor's doing harm since Hippocrates' describes the historical catastrophe of medicine which never been so excitingly and stirringly told.

A large number of Anthropological works focused instead on the humanistic dimension of tribal medicine opposing the critical stand taken by Foucault, Illich and others. Some tried to trivialize it by questioning the 'irrational' outlook towards modernization due to their rigidity and faith in tradition and superstitions. But in many of these studies the socio-political and economic aspects have been grossly ignored with an over emphasis of the cultural descriptions and the role of the supernatural. This trend could be due to the dominance of the world order in which the 'other culture' is a part of the administrative ideology of the colonial and neo-colonial forces.

The Anthropology of illness, influenced by hermeneutically oriented Anthropology of Symbolism, has focused on the cognitive and symbolic dimensions of illness. Good (1977), who collected case histories from Turkik speaking people of Iran and also from an out-patient clinic in the United States, for example, developed the notion of the 'semantic illness network' which he defined as the 'network of words, situations, symptoms and feeling which are associated with an illness and give it meaning for the sufferer'. Kleinman (1980) mentions 'explanatory models of illness' which were models of reality and models for purposive action. Blumenhagen (1980, 1981) also described semantic illness net works to explain how hypertension was perceived by some American patients related to its causes and effects. The Anthropology of sickness, on the other hand, focuses on the social relations, which 'produce the forms and distribution of sickness in society' (Young, 1982). This approach concentrates not on illness experience, but on social systems, power structures, and the social meaning and outcome of sickness.

Each society possesses its own set of rules for the transition of signs into symptoms, the definition of illness and the patterns of treatment. Social forces not only affect diagnosis but also the access to different kinds of therapists and their treatment by different sectors of the population. At the same time, medical practices are also ideological practices, since, as Young notes, 'symbols of healing are simultaneously symbols of power' (Seymour-smith, 1986).

Young (1982) suggested a schematized outline of Medical Anthropology and its fields:

1. Biological Orientation:
   (a) Bio-medicine
   (b) Anthropology of diseases (Biological Anthropology)
2. Socio-cultural orientation:
   (a) Empiricist epistemologies:
      1. Medical Sociology
      2. Empiricist Medical Anthropology
   (b) Non-empiricist epistemologies:
      1. Traditional Anthropological approaches
      2. Anthropology of Illness
      3. Anthropology of sickness

Clinical Anthropology, a branch of Medical Anthropology, may be distinguished here whose primary objective is to increase clinical efficiency, from the type of Medical Anthropology that is concerned with the analysis of social power relations and the production of medical knowledge. Clinical Anthropology incorporates cross-cultural sensitivity into medical practice and encourages awareness of the patient's cognitive-symbolic organization of the experience of sickness and healing. In the wake of such studies, identification of different medical systems in different cultural systems was made possible, rendering critical evaluation of our own systems against such a background more meaningful.

Earlier Studies

Medical Anthropological data were collected from three different sources (Bhasin and Srivastava, 1991:8). Physical Anthropology collected data related to evolution, adaptation, comparative anatomy, racial types, genetics and serology, genetics and environment, and their relation to sickness. The Culture and Personality school of 1930s and 40s was another source for data collection. Such data collected by psychiatrists and anthropologists (Hallowell, 1940, 1963; Henry and Henry, 1944; Paul, 1950) were primarily theoretical in nature with less applied value. The ethnographers collected details about primitive medicine, witchcraft, sorcery and magic. These accounts of beliefs and practices were based on conceptualization of disease as the product of indigenous cultural viewpoint and not in the conceptual framework of modern medicine.

Rivers (1924) dealt with some basic concepts, especially the idea that indigenous medical systems are social institutions and they should be studied in the same way as social institutions are studied. Further, he states that the local medical practices are rational and they should be understood in the context of their own culture. Rivers maintained that religion, magic, and medicine are interrelated, and should be studied in relation to one another, which is still a guiding point for those working on the relatively isolated communities.

Evans-Pritchard's(1937) significant contribution on Azande's witchcraft highlights native thinking on a phenomenon that was considered a cause for many unfortunate conditions, illness being one of them. The Azande believe that some people are born witches with a blackish hairy object, locally called *mangu,* under the sternum and by virtue of their inherent quality they can cause any misfortune. The affected persons fall sick and eventually may die. Witchcraft provides a natural philosophy for explaining misfortunes. Evans-Pritchard describes medical beliefs and practices using a conceptual framework, which was intended for studying other aspects of social structure, such as maintenance of orderly social relations.

Fabrega Jr, (1972) has done an impressive survey of literature related to medical anthropology. His review falls under the categories of, general works, ethno-medical studies, medical ecology and epidemiology. Prominent among the general works are Lieban's (1967) Cebuano sorcery among the Philippines and Blums (1965) depiction of illness and medical care experiences with reference to social processes and traditions in rural communities of Greece. Harwood (1970) studied disease and death among the Safwa people of East Africa to explain the social phenomena of witchcraft and sorcery related to illness and death. Reed (1966) analyzed the influence of socio-cultural and environmental factors on health problems among the pre-literate groups. The German historian Vogel (1970) reviewed American Indian medical beliefs, theories, practices, and therapeutics. Kiev (1968) studied folk psychiatry with an intention to examine how cultural factors affect the form and content of Mexican–American folk medical theories and treatment.

Ethnomedical studies generally deal with medical beliefs, illness descriptions, context of medical problems and medical care, medical treatment, personal characteristics of the medical practitioner, etc., Khare (1963), for example, studied the medical beliefs of the people of Indian villages and how they were linked to contrasting medical systems. His study focused on the influence of those beliefs on the implementation of modern medical programmes. Opler's (1963) account of illness in rural Uttar Pradesh in India followed the theme of the social and moral basis of illness emphasizing the point that medical beliefs are constituents of the general philosophy of the culture. Fabrega (1970, 1971) elaborately dealt with the relations between native conceptual traditions about illness and Western scientific medical knowledge, drawing upon data related to Zinacantan Maya of Chiapas.

Under illness descriptions, Newman's (1964) description of 'wild man' behaviour in New Guinea, Langness's (1965) accounts related to western psychiatric principles, and Rubel's (1964) analysis of the history and distribution of *susto* illness in Hispanic America, are note worthy. There are several other significant studies by Koch (1968), Hoskin et al (1969), Freed and Freed (1864), Lewis (1966), Wilson (1967) and a host of others. Ethnomedical descriptions of illness features and illness classification, the moral, social, and interpersonal dimensions are generally given emphasis in all these studies.

Some of the significant studies related to contexts of medical care include Shiloh' (1965) study which presented a case study among Hausa of northern Nigeria contrasting the native beliefs and orientations toward leprosy with those of Christian missionaries who had attempted to treat leprosy and by depicting how competing medical traditions can interact in a positive way to control a prominent health problem; Press's (1969) study in Bagota, Colombia, contains a very useful analysis of the patterns and implications of dual use of medical systems including a sensitive awareness of the expressive factors that play a role in the use of medical care facilities and personnel.

The treatment of illness received a great deal of attention in the literature. Frank's (1963) analysis of factors that play a role in the modification of behaviour by social and interpersonal factors in such diverse situations as religious conversion, psychotherapy, curing ceremonies is a classic. His account on religious healing contains a number of excellent insights including a discussion of the probable physiological consequences of curing ceremonies that can affect health status. Kennedy's (1967) work deals more directly with psychological illnesses while Osborne (1969) studied the village psychiatric treatment among the Yoruba people.

Studies dealing with shamanistic medical practitioners generally have focused on personality attributes and more specifically on the health status of shamans viewed from a psychological stand point. Margetts (1965) extensively reviewed the practices of the traditional Yoruba healers stressing the personalistic motivations and intentions of the healers. Tenzel (1970) studied the characteristics of shamans, including the basis of their curing powers and their assumptions about health and illness, and the relation of shamanism to the iilness, *susto*.

According to Fabrega Jr (1972:189), "to a very large extent topics dealt with in ethnomedicine have not been subject to precise definition, systematization, testing, subsequent refinement, and elaboration, which, in time, leads to the accumulation of knowledge valuable to anthropology". He further states that Anthropology stands to gain by developing a behavioral framework for examining illness.

Numerous studies in the area of health and illness were undertaken by Indian Anthropologists in different parts of the country, mostly among the tribal populations. Some of the recent publications include number of edited books. Basu (1994) edited an excellent collection of papers on varied topics related to health and illness, like, 'perceptions of health and patterns of health seeking behaviour', 'social, cultural and environmental factors of tribal health', 'food, nutrition and physical growth', 'traditional tribal medicine and modern health care system', 'approaches to health development', etc., Notable contributors to this volume include, Mahapatra, Sachidananda, Bhupender Singh, Buddhadeb Chaudhari, Tandon, B.M.Das, Malhotra, S.C. Tiwari, etc.,

Singh and Mahanti (1995) examined the traditional health care in retrospect and recommended an integrated system of modern and traditional medicine. They also discussed specific diseases afflicting tribals, tribal genetics, tribal and traditional medicine, family planning and welfare, health care and delivery systems.

Hiramani (1997) documented the cultural correlates of tribal health covering four states in India. He studied 1642 tribal households drawn from 16 tribal groups from Andhra Pradesh, 8 from Gujarat, 4 and 10 from Maharashtra and Orissa respectively. His work suggested that the cultural attributes of the tribals have great influence on some aspects of health while external factors on other aspects.

Mutharayappa (2000) studied tribal fertility, morbidity and health care practices among Jenu kuruba and Kadu kuruba tribes inhabiting the hilly and forest areas of the state Karnataka. Roy Burman's (2003) work on six villages and a few small towns in Sikkim, including the capital city Gangtok, deals with the extent of dependence of different medical practices and examines the recent changes affecting the health care scenario in Sikkim. Kalla and Joshi (2004) edited a collection of papers under the title,' Tribal health and medicine'.

The Fundamental Nature of Medical Anthropology

Based on our assumptions about health and illness it is often assumed that others, while they may differ on particulars, fundamentally hold the same views as us about the broader value of identifying, diagnosing and managing the health problems which ourselves perceive to exist. Through detailed anthropological study this often turns out not to be the case. Not only many people fail to identify similar health problems to ourselves, but may identify a range of others, which we would not consider as health problems at all. These views may be based on quite different views about who people are, how their communities and their own bodies operate, where they have come from, what their life objectives should be, and the part that some thing similar to what we call 'health' plays a key role in meeting those objectives. Despite apparently being immersed in scientific approaches to understanding the world these developing countries where, at first sight, a different 'culture' is more immediately obvious. Indeed who we are is a matter of intense cultural debate, as many different peoples exist together in industrialized societies, with many different patterns of health beliefs and behaviours. Thus understanding who both we and others are in this situation involves examining our own beliefs as much as those of others, and making 'the familiar strange'. Further, to understand why people have the health beliefs and behavious that they do, involves studying the whole not just part of their lives. In addition a number of anthropological concepts and perspectives go into the basic orientations of Medical Anthropology.

Concepts and Perspectives

Anthropological perspectives and concepts related to the study of health and disease are built into the orientations of Medical Anthropology. It becomes therefore, necessary to understand some of the important Anthropological concepts applied in Medical Anthropology.

Emic and Etic Perspectives

These terms were originally coined by the linguist Kenneth Pike in 1967 and derived from the words 'phonemic' and 'phonetic'. Phonetic accounts of language are based on the observer's measurement of physical sound differences, while phonemic accounts are those based on speaker's conscious or unconscious models of sound differences. The distinction between *emics* and *etics* in Anthropology became popular for a time, used for the contrast between the explication and presentation of indigenous models of reality on the one hand and the description and comparison of socio-cultural systems according to the observer's criteria on the other. *Emic* analyses are, therefore, those which stress the subjective meanings shared by a social group and their culturally specific model of experience, while *etic* analysis refers to the development and application of models derived from the analyst's theoretical and formal categories. This contrast is linked to the debate about 'cultural relativism' and opposing positions in Anthropology. However, it is generally recognized that the *emic/etic* distinction is not one that can be too straightforwardly employed in Anthropology, since what distinguishes the discipline is precisely its combination of different kinds of 'native models', including the observer's own native models derived from his culture and society, with a different kind of attempt at theoretical synthesis or generalization. The *emic/etic* distinction, while it cannot be used to classify or divide anthropological approaches into neat categories, nevertheless points to a crucial area of controversy and of great theoretical importance within the discipline. However, this anthropological perspective made other social scientists realize the significance of *emic* data collection to occupy a large part of their qualitative research strategy. The concept *emic* basically refers to the data that reflect the native's point of view, where as the *etic* refers to the language and categories of the researchers, 'the out side' biomedical ways of conceptualizations of health and disease. The *emic* perspective is widely used in the area of health and disease while studying the native or tribal cultures. In fact, medical anthropology indulges in the construction of illnesses in terms of native cultures, i.e., from the native's point of view which is the *'emic'* perspective.

Cultural Relativism

The proponents of this theory are the students and followers of Franz Boas in North America. In the works of Boas and many of his students, there was a reaction against 19th century evolutionist theory or 'speculative history' in favour of a *Historical Particularistic* approach, which stressed the need for careful and holistic study of each culture's unique features as an antidote to premature evolutionary generalizations. The growth of Anthropological fieldwork tradition, later strengthened by the 'participant observation method' of Malinowski and the emerging Structural-functionalist School in British Anthropology, led to an increased emphasis on the systemic nature of other cultures and other societies. This has focused on the need for Anthropologist as ethnographer to penetrate the inner logic and inner realty of that worldview and social system. Thus, Anthropologists on both sides of the Atlantic assumed the defense of indigenous and peasant peoples against the 'ethnocentric' and 'racist' assumptions of much 19th century Anthropology, and assumed it under the banner of 'cultural relativism' arguing that each culture or each society possessed its own rationality and coherence in terms of which its customs and beliefs were to be interpreted. This point, endorsing emicist approach, is amply reflected in works related to ethno-medicine in different traditional societies of the world.

Cultural Ecology

A rich body of 'health data related to ecological factors is another significant contribution of Anthropologists. Ecologically oriented Anthropologists tend to view environment as a complex system of interacting groups or populations of different plant and animal species living under a limited range of geological and climatic conditions. A human society is regarded as just another group or species within this complex ecosystem. Human society has to adapt to environmental challenges: to physical and chemical factors in the environment, to the presence of other species, and to the threat posed by other subgroups of the same species. Alland (1966,1970) conducted anthropological studies of disease and illness with an ecological framework.

Cultural adaptation presupposes that man is capable of learning and that he grows up in a human society. Culture is not just the sum of individual behaviours; it is the shared and symbolically transmitted knowledge that is used for interpreting, exploiting, and responding to the environment. On the individual level, humans adapt to changes in the environment by morphological adjustments and acclimatizations. The goal of adaptation is homeostasis within each system and subsystem. A system is in homeostasis if it can maintain its internal composition within certain limits. A human population remains in homeostasis if natality, and morbidity do not seriously threaten its internal complexity and diversity. Homeostasis can be easily upset by interventions originating outside the system, which may bring in new genes, new foods, new ideas, new tools, and new parasites. Even minor and well intended interventions, such as introduction of un-iodized table salt or of non-fortified skim milk have been known to upset previous nutritional adaptations, with serious clinical consequences (Bunce 1972). Traditional societies are often the target of such interventions. They have to deal not only with the introduction of new cultural elements but also with the destruction or replacement of others.

In the field of Medicine, the specialists or the native healers, and the native medicines administered are important areas carved out by the Anthropologists. Healers include the doctors and his supporting staff, the local mid-wife, the priest, the native medicine man/magician, the shaman etc., and the medicines administered by the local medicine man is dealt with under popular literature as ethno-medicine, ethno-botany, native medicine, traditional medicine etc.,

The Native Healers

Rich documentation on the native medicine man in different varieties of cultures is made possible by Anthropological researches. Among the native healers the 'shaman' is the most popular. Harper (1957), Opler (1958), Freed and Freed (1979), Jilek (1971), Rahmann (1959), Eliade (1974), Rajpramukh 1976 & 2005) and many others documented spirit possession and the role of shaman in warding off the spirits. In Eastern Ghats the shaman is called *yejjodu, goragadu goravagadu, guruvulu* etc. Explanations offered in the domain of health and disease, according to Anthropologists, are of two kinds viz., scientific and divinatory. The native's explanation of the etiology of diseases invariably is divinatory in nature i.e., tracing the causes to some divine wrath. The shaman appeases the angry gods and goddesses to restore the health by warding off the spirits. Levi-Strauss placed the role of shaman in the upkeep of social order very cogently, "where as a psychoanalytic cure is based upon the patient's recovery of his individual myth, constructed with his elements from the past, the cure in shamanism is predicted on the patient's receiving the social myth from his collective tradition. The collective myth used by the shaman does not correspond to the patient's personal state but reintegrates his alienating experience of sickness within a meaningful whole. Chapter VII gives an elaborate account on the Shaman.

Ethno-Medicine

Studies in this area focus on non-western medical systems and the beliefs and practices other than those embodied in conventional allopathic 'scientific' medicine. A number of Anthropological studies dealt with the general beliefs and definitions of illness. Khare(1963) dealt with medical beliefs held by Gopalpur villagers and stressed the fact that these beliefs quite often link with contrasting medical systems. Some ethno-medical studies have dealt with the functional role of traditional medicines in particular cultures, others have emphasized the logic behind ethno-medicines; some others have offered the psychological and psycho-somatic implications of these medicines (Bhasin and Srivastava,1991:9).

Ackernecht (1942a, 1942b, 1943, 1945,1947 and 1971) was a pioneer in the study of ethno-medicine. Tracing the relationship between primitive medicine and patterns of culture, he identified three important aspects: (i) there is not one but numerous different 'primitive medicines"; (ii) The differences between the primitive medicines are much less in elements than differences in the medical pattern which they build up and which is culturally contained; and (iii) the degree of integration of different elements of medicine to the whole and of the whole medicine into a cultural pattern varies considerably.

Field researches in different parts of India have yielded a rich body of data on ethno-medicine. Hemadri's (1994) work on the tribal medicine in coastal Andhra districts is a very interesting and significant contribution.

The Methods of Medical Anthropology

Medical anthropologists have traditionally worked through ethnographic methods, that is through spending a lengthy period of time living with a relatively small group of people observing them and recording their way of life as they understand and explain them. Such an approach is increasingly being used in relation to people in industrialized societies, including for example those giving and receiving health care. This approach is time consuming, but social-cultural anthropologists maintain that it is necessary and essential to obtain an account which reflects the daily lives of the people, rather than one which is more cursory and runs the risk of either not understanding more subtle and cyclical beliefs and behaviours, or perhaps more problematically imposing external assumptions and values. However in the light of the resources and time involved in this process a number of more rapid techniques are being used by the skilled ethnographers. RRA (rapid rural appraisal) and a number of other related techniques (PRA) are currently being tested to seek to ensure that key values of the traditional approach can be retained.

Helman (2001:265) suggested new research methods in Medical Anthropology. He delineated four levels of data viz.,

1. What people say they believe, think or do
2. What people actually do

3. What people really think or believe
4. The context of the above three points

According to him the major influences on data collection are:

1. The attributes of the researcher
2. The attributes of the research technique
3. The context in which research takes place

"The implications of this are that, in some cases, different researchers, even when using the identical questionnaires, may produce very different data from the same population. Often this is due to some subtle influence of their personal attributes such as age, gender, ethnicity, dress, body language, tone of voice, religions or political background and so on, on the people being interviewed (Helman 2001: 265). Similarly the presence of a Video Camera or a tape reader may influence the interview process. People behave differently in different contexts and the same Questionnaire administered may produce varied responses depending on the context.

Ethnographic data are now being collected in a relatively shorter period of time instead of spending more than a year's time in the name of participant observation. These new techniques are becoming popular as they are regarded particularly useful in the planning, design and evaluation of health education, disease prevention, and international aid programmes. "They are particularly relevant in situations where research (and policy decisions to be based on that research) need to be fairly close together in terms of time. This is the case in situations of emergency (such as refugee crisis or natural disasters) or in outbreaks of infections diseases, where rapid control can save many lives, especially among the young, elderly and vulnerable. Traditional fieldwork or ethnography which can take up to 2-3 years to complete, write up and analysis is simply not useful in this type of situation" (Helman, 2001: 263).

2

INDIGENOUS KNOWLEDGE

Indigenous knowledge research is a recent trend in the sociological and Anthropological domains. Hither to fore, all developmental programmes initiated especially by the Government agencies have adopted a top-down approach, i.e., planning, distribution, and resources in-flow and perceptions flow from top to down. This trend has been recently reversed with a growing realization that for any successful implementation of planned programme, people's participation becomes imperative. In this context, participatory research techniques have been generated in different social sciences. The main thrust in such an approach is to make the people or the subjects into active collaborators in bringing about desired change. In this background research on Indigenous knowledge systems is growing steadily and anthropological contributions in this area have been greatly acknowledged, as the basic research methodology adopted by Anthropologists is participant observation method. In fact, the pioneers in documenting indigenous knowledge systems all over the world, especially among the less advanced, disadvantaged tribal and rural masses were none other than the Anthropologists. In the area of health and disease too, many anthropologists have undertaken documentation of health-related issues

Nonetheless, explanations offered in this domain are mostly divinatory in nature implying the divine wrath as causative of all diseases. In this paper, an attempt is made to illustrate the health status of the Tribals of Eastern Ghats and their health seeking behaviour and beliefs. Despite the fact that tribal societies exhibit similarities in many aspects related to health and disease, local variations persist.

The study of indigenous knowledge is a new revolution set in the domain of Anthropology. In its wake, this new knowledge interface has created a new awareness on the part of Anthropologists to critically look at their conventional methodological armour. Indigenous knowledge deals with a variety of hybrid studies borne out of a battle of different perspectives, leading to a critique of our understanding of knowledge as such. A holistic perspective on human knowledge would help us understand the implications of indigenous knowledge especially in the areas of health and disease. In this context, of late, Anthropologist's ability to facilitate incorporation of indigenous knowledge into development process has assumed greater significance.

Knowledge and the Development of Indigenous Knowledge

An ideal system of knowledge is generally seen as one that derives its corpus from abstract principles by systematic deduction. Modern academic knowledge is 'a way of knowing' that emerged historically through the union of a number of ideas which are subjected to global systematization through "centers of calculation", nurturing its spectacular accumulation, scope and power (Latour, 1987).

Such an understanding is questioned with the advent of the recognition of indigenous knowledge as a living and dynamic tacit knowledge interfacing with an all encompassing human activity in all societies, which "scientific knowledge is not always capable of validating' (Brouwer, 1999). The heretical idea gained currency that 'other' people have their own effective 'science' and resource use practices and to assist them we need to understand their knowledge and management systems and "those others" may have something to teach us (Atte, 1992; Barrow, 1992; Fairhead, Rajasekaran, Warren & Babu, 1991).

In his exploration of the ethnography of human knowledge, Barth (2002) maintains that "knowledge in its different modalities can range from an assemblage of disconnected empirical detail to a 'theory of everything'... as we are in a world constructed on principles of sociality and morality, not mechanical causality". Indigenous knowledge is explained as "local, orally transmitted, a consequence of practical engagement reinforced by experience, empirical rather than theoretical, repetitive, fluid and negotiable, shared but asymmetrically distributed, largely functional, and embedded in a more encompassing cultural matrix, that which is not epitomized by being a part of a dominant Western scientific knowledge" (Ellen and Harris, 1997). By definition, Indigenous knowledge research is a "small scale, culturally specific and geographically localized, infrequently encompassing regional ecosystems" (Sillitoe, 1998). This position highlights the centrality of localized socio–cultural context in understanding and appreciating indigenous knowledge.

Barth (2002) presents an analytical framework to distinguish three components of knowledge viz. substantive corpus of assertions, a range of media representation and a social organization. He demonstrates that all the three are interconnected and appear together in particulars of action, in every transaction in knowledge, in every performance. In this context, the tribal cosmology, rituals and religious traditions fall within this concept of knowledge. These traditions also provide the people with a world-view and to act accordingly. They encompass aspects of nature and cosmos, health and life, ethno psychology, human morality and a panoply of supernatural entities that erratically affect and may even invade and possess human beings.

Tribal Ethno-medicine as a Science

With the advent of indigenous knowledge perspective, there is a radical shift in the mind set from viewing native systems of thought as naive and rudimentary, even savage to a recognition that local cultures know their plant, animal and physical resources intimately (Nazarea, 1999). If we reflect on the idea that traditional ethno-medicine as science, we must ask how this can be so: scientific principles are constructed through scientific theory and practice where as tribal healing is rooted in the latent knowledge structures and livelihood practices of local people. Both kinds of knowledge are grounded in social practice but very different kinds of practice, based on different categories and assumptions, involving particular experiences, values and cultural definitions.

Atran (1999) maintains that indigenous knowledge structures are like scientific theories in that they generalize from concrete experience, but unlike theories they are not systematic formulations of laws or methods. Rather, they involve the adjustment of forms of human livelihood to the environment in which they are embedded. The idea that indigenous knowledge must be science because it leads to empirical results consistent with Western Science is based on a concept of nature as a "pre given" and "science" as the only means of discovering its universal laws (Berlin, 1992). However, the nature itself is not perceptually 'given' but 'constructed', in the microscope or in the forest, by 'perceptually guided action', the practices that make up our experience (Nigh, 2002; Varela, Thomson and Rosch, 1991). Attempting to force indigenous knowledge into the mould of "scientific principles" is to reduce an objective reality independent of human experience.

Tambiah (1990) attests that, in reality, rather than an empirical 'folk' science conforming to universal principles of 'real' science, what we have is multiple contrasting orderings of reality. People construct their worlds by their knowledge and live by it, and therefore an Anthropology of knowledge should ask how these varieties are variously produced, represented, transmitted and applied.

Indigenous Knowledge and New Applied Anthropology

Indigenous knowledge research sets out explicitly to make connections between local peoples understanding and practices and those of out side researchers and development workers, notably in the natural resources and health sectors, seeking to achieve a sympathetic and in-depth appreciation of their experience and objectives and to link them to scientific technology (Sillitoe, 1998). In this context, participatory research techniques have been generated in different social sciences and the main thrust in such an approach is to make the people or the subjects into active collaborators in bringing about desired change. Technology transfer is now considered not as a top–down imposition but as a search for jointly negotiated advances, which results in cost-effective, time-effective programmes generating appropriate insights readily intelligible even to non-experts. Thus participatory approaches seek a more systematic accommodation of indigenous knowledge in research and technological interventions (Schaffer, 1989). The demands of indigenous knowledge and participatory research require the establishment of partnerships founded on dialogue. Anthropologists are better positioned to take up the tasks of incorporating indigenous knowledge into the development process, as they are the pioneers in documenting indigenous knowledge systems through participant observation method that involves living with the subjects for a very long period. This being the hallmark of Anthropological research, the role-play of 'Anthropologists as consultants' in implementing development programmes becomes much more relevant compared to other social scientists.

Haile (1996) proposes that the idea of harnessing Anthropology to technical knowledge to facilitate development puts the discipline where it should be, at the center of the development process. This focus on indigenous knowledge has already resulted in reappraising theoretical as well as methodological aspects of Anthropology. The liability of indigenous knowledge is reflected in the theoretical shift from a structural to a processual and to a post-modernist perspective. Certain methodological advances to tailor interventions to local conditions have already been put forward by the Anthropologists in 'doing Anthropology' by a very different process.

The process involves the brokering of knowledge in which Anthropologists become researchers for and consultants to indigenous people and traditional communities (community-controlled research). They can also oversee that the indigenous knowledge is not patented for but used in the production of universal medical technologies, not for private commercial benefits. This will establish the 'dialogue' as the cornerstone of a new Applied Anthropology. In this endeavour, the greatest challenge to Anthropology vis-à-vis development debate is to develop criteria and indicators for sustainable development–health environments, sustainable livelihoods that are based on local, indigenous perceptions, classifications, values, measures of environmental quality and change that reflects local observations and knowledge systems, even if they seem 'magical', whimsical or destructive to the outsider.

The Cultural Logic of Tribal Medicine in Eastern Ghats

Eastern Ghats in South India are a long chain of broken hills and mountain ranges spread over three states, Orissa, Andhra Pradesh and Tamil Nadu. These Eastern Ghats are inhabited by a number of tribes and of the 33 scheduled tribes in Andhra Pradesh, 22 live in Eastern Ghats. Some of the prominent tribes of North Coastal Andhra Pradesh are, the *Bagata, Gadaba, Jatapu, Savara, Konda Dora, Khond, Valmiki* etc. Tribal religion is mostly animistic although the influence of Hinduism is seen in some religious practices. Invoking divine beings for blessings is a common practice at the time of agricultural operations. In the area of health too, dependence on divinatory forces is distinctly visible in their curative practices.

In many tribal societies knowledge related to these aspects is treated as esoteric and is associated with certain specialized roles, inherited by certain people, most notably, the shaman. The medicine man or shaman is called as *Yejjodu* among the *Savara* and *Jatapu, Guruvulu* or *Guru* among the *Bagatha, Konda Dora* and *Valmiki, Vijjodu* among the *Koya, Vaidyadu* among the *Konda Reddy*. Just as supernatural wrath casts its spell occasionally in the form of varieties of illnesses, the shaman looks at the cure for these illnesses as located in the very supernatural beings that cause them. Thus, the etiology of the disease and the cure of the disease are located in the same source, i.e., the supernatural. The shamans are powerful stewards in a symbolic and metaphysical domain which is central to 'supernaturalism' of the tribal communities. By supernatural favour, the shaman is believed to possess the gift of healing as well as the knowledge about medicinal plants.

The shaman treats disease essentially by religious means, through sacrifice and prayer. Herbs have healing power because of the prayers recited and rituals performed by the shaman. The etiology of sickness varies–human intention and behaviour, either of the patient or of others in the patient's life-world, result of deviant behaviour, disrespect towards elders and refusal to meet obligations of reciprocity with neighbours and relatives etc., Misdemeanor results in soul loss or illness. Also, economic or other success or refusal to share good fortune provokes envy and sorcery among neighbours. Etiology, diagnosis, treatment and prognosis among the tribals of Eastern Ghats show more similarities than variations.

The curing ceremonies are 'socially reconstituting and reoriginating' (Kapferer, 1996). The shaman seeks to restore the patient's relationship to the physical, metaphysical and social worlds–to correct the imbalance that is the root cause of illness. The recovery of good health and good relationship with fellow community members is achieved by one or more curing ceremonies.

Unlike the linear cure-for-disease equation of modern (allopathic) medicine, the local medicine practiced by shamans (Harper 1957) who use herbs is located in a more complex 'socially reconstituting and reorganising' context. Shamans base their practices on holistic epistemologies of illness and curing handed down through generations (Rajpramukh 1976; Kakar 1982). In their therapeutic interventions, shamans seek to manipulate the bodily, spiritual and social domains at once. They do not sharply dichotomize between organic and supernatural causes of disease–all sickness has both aspects, though in varying degrees, and both aspects must be treated if the patient is to be cured. The Valmiki *Guruvulu* (shaman) maintains that the herbs are useful, but it is the confession of misbehaviour and repentance is what really cures the patients.

The ethnography of a wide variety of tribal communities in the Eastern Ghats in general suggests a native cosmology in which the notions related to metaphysical balance is a key concept. It is the belief that "continued human existence is predicated on the maintenance of cyclic cosmic balance that both affects and reflects earthly conditions" in terms of "harmony between the physical and metaphysical worlds" (Fischer, 1999: 480).

Indigenous Knowledge of the Tribals

The Diagnostic Procedures and Techniques of Shamans among different tribes of Eastern Ghats present many similarities. Whenever evil spirits possesses any person, the person's pulse becomes very weak and his/her hands become cold as ice and the patient appears restless. The first step the Shaman takes is to place a winnow containing burnt cow dung cake over the head of the patient. He inscribes the name of a popular god on this cow dung ash. Then invoking the name of his Guru, he chants some mantras to propitiate his spirit-familiar. Thus he commissions his sprit-familiar into the ash which now becomes sacred powder (*vibhoothi*) and smears it on the forehead of the patient. Then he takes a handful of this sacred powder and blows it over the head of his patient. Immediately the evil spirit leaves the patient and the patient regains full consciousness. If the spirit still refuses leave the patient, the shaman mixes pepper powder with the juice extracted from *Tulasi* leaves and smears it on the eyes of the patient. This medication causes burning sensation in the eyes and tears roll down the eyes of the patients relieving the spirit too. In this haunted condition the patient also would be able to reveal the name of the spirit when his little finger's nail is pressed hard.

If the sickness is due to sorcery or witchcraft, the shaman performs a prayer to invoke his spirit-familiar and decides the course of treatment. It is also believed that the spirits of the dead ancestors also appear in the dreams of either the patient or the shaman and are informed of the mode of treatment to be followed.

The shamans in this region also use talismans. They tie them around their neck of upper hand, even after warding off the evil spirits, to protect their patients from a relapse of ghost haunting.

To know whether the patient is affected by ghosts, spirits etc., they make the patient smell a dried herb *'Adavi Pasupu'*. If the patient feels no smell, it is believed that a ghost affected the patient. But if he feels a pungent and foul smell, he is considered normal and healthy. They, then use "*Voocha Kommu*" to throw away the evil spirit.

To know what kind of ghost or evil spirit is acting on a patient, they usually feel the pulse (*nadi*). Some specified parts in the palm have been given names. They hold the wrist of the patient with one hard, and study the points on the palm. At whatever point they feel the change, that point is the ghost, which is said to be responsible for the illness. Then they use the appropriate method to ward off that ghost.

To know the life chances of a person, bitten by a snake, they crush some kinds of leaves in their palms. If, it produces white foam, they believe that the patient would survive, but if only water comes without foam, the patient would, for sure, die.

To detect leprosy, they rub the leaves of *Kodimala* on the suspected area of the body. If the patient feels itchy, the skin is normal, but if the patient feels no itching sensation, the skin is supposed to be infected with leprosy.

Many of the common diseases are treated with the locally available herbs, for example, for cold and cough, a powder made of Devadar bark, and locally called *Pherangi chekka* is used. The powder is mixed with water and is gulped. It is believed that this powder helps in better digestion too.

Similarly for whooping cough, the medicine man ties a *Raksha* (Talisman) around the neck of the child. This Raksha is in the form of a necklace, made out of the fiber of some local tree. If the cough is severe he gives Tuniki Ginga. These seeds have to be crushed into a fine powder and added with some water, made into a fine paste and administered into the child, orally.

For measles, chicken pox etc., the treatment is through the propitiation of local deities. The shaman performs a ritual and uses the flour of chollu, turmeric and some kinds of flowers.

During the ritual he chants mantras in front of the fire and throws *Sambrani* (Frankincense) into it. The smoke that emanates is diverted to the body of the patient and is believed to give relief.

For epidemics, sacrification of goats and chicken is practiced. In case of dog bites and other wounds, that particular bitten area is bound with a rope made of jute and some crushed herbs and medicinal leaves, placed and tied with a cloth.

When a person shows unusual symptoms and changes in behaviour and becomes weak gradually in spite of other curative measures, the people believe that he is affected with the *Dumba* (evil spirit). The medicine man possesses innate powers and based on the symptoms identified, a particular ancestor of a spirit is considered responsible for the ill health of the person. Then he follows a procedure to get in to trance to identify the deceased ancestor. That procedure requires materials like "*korra*' flour, *Sindhur*, turmeric power, *sambrani*, eggs and different types of fruits and flowers. He also chants some mantras. If the patient dies in spite of the shaman's efforts, the blame is passed on only to the powerful evil spirits, but not to the shaman.

3

ILLNESS AMONG THE TRIBALS

Anthropological research in health and illness is a relatively recent trend despite the fact that a substantial body of beliefs, knowledge and practices in every society is built around the major life experiences of health and illness. Ackernecht (1947) has rightly pointed out: "Disease and its treatment are only in the abstract purely biological processes. Actually, such facts as whether a person gets sick at all, what kind of disease he acquires and what kind of treatment he receives depend largely upon social factors". The significant links between human behaviour and disease etiology and transmission have been recognized for many ,years as illustrated in the works of Alland (1972), Dunn (1976, 1979 and 1983), Hesser (1982), Polgar (1964) and Randy (1978).

III-health is universal human experience. But the distribution of diseases in kind and magnitude varies from society to society and this variance could be explained with the help of different biological, ecological and social-cultural factors. This chapter deals with the distribution of different kinds of diseases among the tribes of Visakhapatnam district in Andhra Pradesh, India.

Alland (1972) studied how cultural practices could be used to promote health and hygiene. Drawing upon the concept form mathematical modeling , he used the term 'minimax' to refer to cultural behaviours that minimize the risk of disease and maximize the health of the groups. However, in case of tribals in India it is found that many of their behavioural practices are not in consonance with this model.

Polgar (1962) in his illuminating paper on health and human behaviour delineated areas of interest common to the social and medical Sciences. Of the literature published in Medical Anthropology, while some papers are exhaustive and critically evaluative, others have pointed out areas of research among the under-developed people. In many studies, specific socio-economic factors have been dealt with by relating them to the etiology and transmission of various diseases. For example, the etiology of rheumatoid arthritis, hypertension and Schizophrenia were related to socio-economic factors in the works of Scotch. Geiger and Mishler respectively. Chen and Cobb examined the relation between family structure and general health. The major criticism such studies elicited was that they have not contributed much towards the general theories of human behaviour. In this context, Kunstadter (1962:185) writes that, "Part of the difficulty... is due to the fact that health is not the same sort of a 'field' in the social sciences as is, for example, the study of political structures, kinship or economics". So the general significance of studies on health and human behaviour largely remain illustrative. Scotch, on the other hand, maintains that these arguments are marginal explanations and it could be argued that poor research is the cause rather than the result of inferior role of social scientists. But the fact remains that researches in this area, whether evaluative or illustrative, are always helpful in furthering our knowledge, especially in designing projects meant for the promotion of health and hygiene among different kinds of people. Report clearly bring out the substantive and methodological gains of an Anthropologists and clinicians. Undoubtedly, the field is inherent with a tremendous scope for inter-disciplinary research.

Socio-cultural factors are important in explaining the etiology, transmission and treatment of a few diseases among some of the tribals of Munchingput Mandal in Visakhapatnam district, in Andhra Pradesh state. The common distribution of diseases and their etiologies among the tribals of Visakhapatnam District is presented here.

Tribals in Visakhpatnam District

The district presents two distinct geographical divisions, the strip of land along the coast and interior called the plains division and the hilly area of eastern ghats on the north and the west, called the agency division. According to 1991 census, the total tribal population of Visakhapatnam district is 5,57,572 distributed over 6,298 square kilometers, of which 2,78,399 are males and 2,79,173 are females. There are 11 mandals in the Revenue division of Paderu, of which Munchingput mandal comprises the largest number of villages (467). The inhabitants of this mandal are predominantly tribals who include Valmikis, Konda Doras, Bagathas, Malis, Porjas etc. With an literacy rate of 16.58% and with a large majority of them still reeling under poverty, most of the tribals still eke out their living primitive means. Shifting cultivation, an age-old practice is still prevalent among them and it is still a major source of their livelihood. Recently a few of them are employed as coolies in road and building construction activity.

Relating illness and illness manifestation to the wrath of evil spirits and gods is an age-old practice in many societies. For example, to the Acadians (2500 BC), if some one becomes ill, it was either his own fault (for having sinned) or the making of outside agents, such as bad smells, cold evil spirits, or goods.

Distribution of Diseases

The total new cases reported during the years 1983 and 86 (4 years) were 1, 83,452 and forms an average of 10.5% of the total population. In other words, about 10% of the total population falls sick every year. The following table gives 10 major diseases among the tribals during 1983-86 with their corresponding prevalence rate.

Prevalence of various diseases among the tribals of Visakhapatnam district during 1983-86:

Type of diseases	*No. of cases Reported*	*Average per year*	*Proportion (%)*
Skin disease	1,69,205	42,301	23.28
Anaemia	1,31,889	32,972	18.14
Arthritis	74,995	18,749	10.32
Malnutrition	72,133	18,033	9.92
Malaria	15,213	3,803	2.09
Eye diseases	10,769	2,692	1.48
Acute respiratory	8,424	2,106	1.16
Peptic ulcer	7.921	1,980	1.09
Ancylostomiasis	7,910	1,978	1.09
Diseases of Teeth	5,036	1,259	0.69
All other diseases	2,23,442	55.861	30.74
Total	7,26,936	1,81,734	100.00

Skin Disease

It tops the list of diseases among the tribals. The most commonly reported skin disease among them is scabies which is caused by the itch mite (*sacoptes scabei*). The female mite burrows into the skin and lays eggs causing intense itching which is usually worse at night. Transmission of mites occurs by close body contact and by infected clothes. Among the tribals, unhygienic habits, lack of adequate water facilities and crowded housing are probably responsible for the spread of infection.

Arthritis

This is another major disease prevalent among the tribals. Osteo-arthritis and Rheumatoid arthritis are most common while gout, tuberculous arthritis and suppurative arthritis are less common among them. Osteo-arthritis is mostly seen in the older age group. This essentially is a 'wear and tear' phenomenon also designated as joint disease characterized by progressive deterioration and loss of cartilage over the years. Rheumatoid arthritis is more prevalent among the females than males, with peak prevalence in 3rd to 4th decades of one's life. It is basically an inflammatory disease of unknown etiology.

Malnutrition

Among the tribals, it is probably due to poverty and ignorance, acute and chronic illness, chronic alchoholism, gastro-intestinal disorders; and diets lacking proteins, vitamin B 12 and iron. Milk consumption is not practiced by the tribals of Visakhapatnam district, which, if adapted, could have had desirable affects on their health status. Of all these factors among the tribals 'alchoholism' is a behavioural factor which assumes significance in the context of malnutrition.

Malaria

It is endemic almost all over India and the tribal areas are not an exception to it. It is caused due to infection with *sporozoan* parasite of the genus *plasmodium* and transmitted to man by infected female *anophelous* mosquito. Open drainages and unhygienic surroundings serve as breeding places for mosquitoes which is the major environmental factor among the tribals too. As a preventive measure, long sleeves and trousers are advocated. But the tribals dress usually covers their private parts only making large parts of their body exposed to mosquito bites. Non–availability of prophylactic drugs also could be another reason for the prevalence of the disease. However, the high incidence of sickle cell among the tribals makes malaria less severe.

Eye Diseases

Of the two eye diseases, trachoma and cataract, trachoma is caused due to the unhygienic conditions. It is a specific communicable kerato conjunctivitis caused by *Chlamydia trachoma*. Transmission is usually by contact or from *fomites* in unhygienic surroundings. Some infections also occur during birth from infected genital passages. Unhygienic surroundings, lack of proper care of the eyes could be easily said to be the causative factors. Lack of trachoma clinics in tribal areas also contributes to the high incidence.

Respiratory Diseases

Some of the respiratory diseases among the tribals are chickenpox, influenza, diphtheria, whooping cough and tuberculosis. These respiratory infections are caused by virus and bacteria. Among many tribals some of these respiratory diseases are caused by excessive alcoholism and smoking.

Peptic Ulcer and other Digestive Disorders

These are usually common in middle aged to older adults. The term 'peptic ulcer' refers to an ulcer in the lower oesophagus, stomach or duodenum. Increased serum levels of calcium stimulate gastrin secretion and therefore acid secretion in the stomach. Patients with peptic ulcer often have a family history of the disease. Individuals of blood group "O" are about 36% more likely to develop these lesions than those of the other blood groups. Males are more susceptible to peptic ulcer. It is caused due to exposure of duodenal mucosa to excessive amounts of acid and peptin and some break down in gastric mucosal defense against acid and peptin. Women are most often affected at, or after, menopause. Smoking usually exacerbates the course of peptic ulcer disease and excessive alcoholism is also bad. The tribal diet, which contains sour gruel and rice beer, may also contribute to the disease.

Ancylostomiasis

It is caused by the hookworm. As hookworms suck blood it results in anaemia. Worm inhabits duodenum and upper jejunum. eggs are passed in stools, hatch in moist soil and produce larvae which can penetrate bare feet and re-infect people. Prevention is by wearing shoes and using latrines. As the tribals defecate in the open and not in the habit of wearing shoes, Ancylostomias spreads unchecked and is one of the major causes of anaemia among the tribals.

Diseases of Teeth

Many of the teeth disorders among the tribals are caused mostly due to their lack of oral hygiene and smoking habits. In addition, it is found that the water that is available in tribal areas lacks such minerals like iodine and fluoride. In such cases supply of iodised salt to the tribals and usage of fluoride toothpastes in general would contain some tooth disorders. This is not practiced by many tribals due to non-availability, lack of awareness and as they are non-customary. The social-cultural factors cited for each disease are only suggestive but not conclusive.

The Yejjodu (shaman)

The belief of the tribals in the existence of such evil spirits and gods is so strong that in the event of disease, their first approach is to local medicine man, the Yejjodu (shaman) who invariably attributes the causes of all diseases to the evil spirits. Raj Pramukh elsewhere described, in details, the role of shaman among the Jatapus. The tribals of Visakhapatnam district in general, and Munchingput mandal in particular believe in the exist-district ence of evil spirits and unless they are appeared, they cannot hope for a cure of their disease. And this appeasement is done only through the shaman.

Many tribals in Munchingput mandal wear a charm around their neck. It immediately indicates that such a person was suffering from some disease and that he was being treated by the shaman. Almost every other kid in tribal villages have this charm around their neck which shows their profound faith in the healing power of shaman. The fees usually collected by the shaman include a bottle or two of native liquor, a hen besides small fees, which varies from Rs. 10 to Rs. 300 depending upon the financial position of the patient. This practice of patronizing the shaman still continues despite the fact that the government opened many primary health centres (P.H.C's) with qualified medical doctors at many places in the tribal areas. It is mostly because of the fear in the tribal mind of the shaman's powers to deal with the evil spirits and engage these to fulfill any of their purposes. The medical officer in the P.H.C. at Muchingput confirmed that many patients are brought into the P.H.C. at a critical stage of the disease; their first approach invariably is to the local shaman. The shaman thus wields enormous influence in the lives of tribals in dealing with sickness.

There was a case of rabies due to dog bite reported at the P.H.C. in 1988. Rabies, also known as hydrophobia (fear of water) is an acute, highly fatal viral infection of the central nervous system. Rabies is generally transmitted to man by the bite of a rabid animal. The virus is inoculated into the skin with the saliva of the biting animal. The saliva may be infective 4 to 5 days before the onset of clinical symptoms. A 13-year-old girl from Munchingput was bitten by a rabid dog and the dog was immediately killed. The girl was brought to the P.H.C. in Munchingput and was given first aid by cleaning and flushing the wound and by administering some antibiotics. The next day, ARV (Anti-rabies vaccine) was brought from Paderu, the Revenue Head quarters, and the girl was treated with ARV for 3 days. Actually this treatment has to be continued for 7-14 days depending on the nature of the wound. Then the girl failed to show up at the PHC for continuation of the ARV and it was later known that she was receiving treatment from the local shaman. After three months, it was reported to the medical doctor at Munchingput that the girl was suffering from rabies apparently due to inadequate immunization. The medical doctor visited the girl in her village, accompanied by a senior assistant and the executive officer. After examining the girl, he confirmed rabies and gave her procaine penicillin. The patient could not take oral medicine as she was already suffering from throat muscle spasms. At that point the shaman came and did not allow the Medical team to shift her to Visakhapatnam General Hospital .The local villages also extended their support to the shaman.

Then the shaman took the girl to the burial ground and the helpless medical team also accompanied them to see what would happen next. Right in their presence, the shaman performed some ritual and when the girl started screaming at the sight of water, even though the medical team was objecting to it, the shaman poured 3 or 4 buckets full of water over the head of the girl. The medical team returned helpless and it was reported later that the girl died next day. This instance clearly attests to the fact that the belief systems of those tribals play a very crucial role in their perception of disease causation and the treatment of disease. For them all diseases are attributed to the evil spirits and the only one capable of warding off the evil spirits is the shaman.

While the belief system influences the perception of disease and accordingly bring in the shaman as much preferred over the modern medicine man, some behavioural practices also contributes to the out break of diseases. For example in Jodiput, inhabited also contributed by Malis, the tribal have a practice of defecating in the open on the hill to, at the bottom of which their villages is located. It is reported by the PHC medical doctor that in this village there is an unusual rate of the incidence of water borne diseases like, gastro–enteritis, amoebiasis, bacillary dysentery and occasionally cholera. It seems during the rainy seasons, the water that flows sown the hill carrying the human faeces is collected in the tank at the bottom of the hill near the village and the same water is being used by tribals for drinking purpose which is the etiological factor for the abnormal rate of water borne diseases among them.

It is also found that sexual behaviour also plays a vital role in the etiology and transmission of diseases. Among many of the tribals, there is a high prevalence of pre-marital and extra-marital relationships. For example among the Porjas of Shrujanapeta, it is reported that young boys of about 13-14 years old indulge in sexual relations even with girls older than their age. It is also reported in some cases that younger boys of 8 or 9 years old also have their own girl friends. In yet another instance, while the sons are still in their tender years, the fathers marry girls on behalf of their sons. While it is beyond the scope of their paper to deal in detail with the marital practices and sexual relations prevalent among these tribals, it becomes necessary here to touch upon some salient features of their sexual life as they pose health problems of unmanageable proportion. It is reported, as the average Porja is drawn into sexual life at an early age and is constantly engaged in it, by the time they reach 30 or 35 years age, they all become old and eventually die at a relatively younger age.

The loose sexual code of conduct among some of the tribals is taken advantage of by the outsiders. For instance, after a battalion of Reserve police were posted in Munchingput to contain the naxalite problem in 1990, there was a rapid increase in the sexually transmitted diseases reported at the Munchingput PHC Problems of this kind could be easily controlled if necessary precautions are taken in checking the contact between tribals and others.

These are but a few instances which bring to light the importance of customary practices and belief systems in the etiology, transmission and treatment of diseases. Their belief in the traditional institutions of shaman, their practices of defecation, their customary sexual behaviours and the advantages take of them by out siders, demonstrate the role of ethological factors in the study of disease and disease manifestation.

4

NUTRITION

Nutrition is a science which studies the relationship between diet and states of health and disease. Dieticians are Health professionals who are specialized in this area of expertise. They are also the only highly trained health professionals able to provide safe, evidence-based and accurate dietary advice and interventions.

Between the extremes of optimal health and death from starvation or malnutrition, there is an array of disease states that can be caused or alleviated by changes in diet. Deficiencies, excesses and imbalances in diet can produce negative impacts on health, which may lead to diseases such as scurvy, obesity or osteoporosis, as well as psychological and behavioral problems. Moreover, excessive ingestion of elements that have no apparent role in health, (e.g. lead, mercury, PCBs, dioxins), may incur toxic and potentially lethal effects, depending on the dose. The science of nutrition attempts to understand how and why specific dietary aspects influence health.

Nutrition is defined as, "combination of processes by which the living organism receives and utilizes the material necessary for the maintenance of its functions for the growth and renewal of its components" (Turner 1959). Malnutrition has been defined as a pathological state resulting from a relative or absolute deficiency or excess of one or more essential nutrients. Under-nutrition is the pathological state resulting from the consumption of inadequate quality food over an extended period of time. Over-nutrition is the pathological state resulting from the consumption of excess quality food and hence a caloric excess over an extended period of time. (WHO, 1966)

The Role of Anthropology

By tradition Anthropologists study small scale societies and in the area of Nutrition they have already made a distinction by their methodology and theories. The holistic approach adapted by Anthropologists helps to assess the nutritional status in relation to other aspects of society.

Since the 1950s data on the nutritional status of various populations have been recorded by different government agencies like the ICMR, NIN etc., and universities as well. In almost all the studies it was recognised poverty as one of the root causes of malnutrition. It may be noted here that 28% of the indian population still lives under poverty. In this context, the need for a paradigm shift was recognised: from food security to nutrition security and from child survival to child health.

Methodology

Anthropologists use number of techniques and tests to collect data related to nutrition and growth. Anthropometry, clinical and bio-chemical tests, assessments on food in-take and functioning of the physical body, vital and health statistics in addition to socio-economic information.

Anthropometry

This technique is used for taking various bodily measurements in the study of nutrition and growth. The measurements for such studies have been listed in the 'Human Biology: A guide to field methods', and certain measure ments like, height, body weight, MUAC, head and chest circumferance from 'IBP Handbook No.9(2)' are useful.A set of 18 measurements have been recommended for a thorough assessment, monitoring and surveillance. Although the Anthropometric instruments seem to be simple the researchers need adequate training in using the appropriate instruments, accurate skills, good recording methods while taking measurements. Statistical calculations and interpretations of various indices produced by these measurements like the BMI (body mass index) have to be cautiously handled, otherwise, a 'normal' individual may end up as being classified as 'malnourished' (Kulkarni, 2005).

In the literature on nutrition a comprehensive list of physical signs associated with nutritional deficiency is invariably given. These are useful in assessing the nutritional status in clinical situation. But examination of such signs does not reveal the extent of depletion. In addition, due to inaccuracy in personal examination there are likely to be individual variations.

Biochemical Variations

In the Cambridge Encyclopedia of Human Growth and development a number of biochemical tests have been mentioned but most of them are suitable only for the laboratory but not suitable for field-based studies.

Assessment of Food Intake

A number of methods of food analysis are available such as weigh as you eat; 24 hour recall method and so on. Every method has both some advantages and disadvantages and as per the requirements any convenient method could be adopted. For the caloric estimation and the consumption of a particular nutrient or micronutrient these methods prove to be very useful. Administration of schedules or questionnaires is more suitable techniques to collect data.

Health Statistics

Data related to fertility, mortality and morbidity are very useful to draw valid conclusions and generalizations. Primary data related to these vital statistics throw light on the factors related to infant/child and maternal mortality.

Socio-Economic Conditions

Data related to various socio-economic factors are very useful as they influence human life in various ways and this body of information also helps in interpreting data related to nutrition.

Functional Assessment

It is related to the functioning of bodily parts. In addition to the Bio-chemical assessment, the examination of the condition of RBC's, strength or weaknesses of nerves, of blood vessels, the capacity of the body to function efficiently, heart beats, the functioning of all other systems is included in this type of assessment.

Evaluation of Nutrition involves all these techniques and methods. All these things have to be critically considered as they basically work out to be a holistic approach. Appropriate methods have to be carefully applied depending on the context. While dealing with the nutrition status of refugees and displaced populations (SHERE project) the World Health Organization has given the following list of a number of prerequisites in the nutritional assessment:

1. The concept, theories and methodologies of child growth be understood,
2. The level of body composition such as atomic, molecular, cellular, tissue system and whole body be clear,
3. The measurements, indices, indicators be clearly understood. A valid nutritional indicator owes a substantial proportion of its variability of differences in nutrition. For any given indicator, however, this proportion may vary across or within populations. BMI for example is a good indicator of variability in energy reserves in individuals with a sedentary life style; but not in athletes,
4. For identification of individuals or populations at risk the indicator must reflect past and present risk and predict the future risk,
5. For selection of individuals or populations for an intervention the indicator must predict the benefit to be derived from the intervention,

6. Evaluation of the effects of changing nutritional, health or socio-economic influences, including interventions the indicator must reflect response to the past and present,
7. Interventions,
8. Excluding individuals from high risk treatments, from employment or from certain benefits, and
9. Assessing achievements of normative standards indicator must reflect 'normality'.

Nutritional Deficiency Diseases

We need food for energy, growth and maintenance and also for protection. When the right kinds of foods are not taken the body fails to grow and function normally. This leads to various diseases.

Protein Energy Malnutrition

This is a common deficiency disease in India. The first sign of malnutrition among the children is failure to gain weight and much worse is loss of weight. Diarrhoea and other diseases also make the condition still worse.

During the first 6 months after the birth, when children are breastfed, they grow well. After that weight gain stops and breast-feeding has to be complemented with other suitable foods. If this is not done, weight gain will stop and the child becomes prone to various diseases. Some of the early signs of malnutrition include: the muscles look wasted and the child looks thin; the belly looks prominent; the child is listless and does not respond when the mother plays with him; the child looks short for his age; and the hair looks light or reddish instead of dark. To put short, failure to gain weight every mouth is an early sign of malnutrition. The child becomes normal with simple treatment at this stage.

Marasmus and Kwashiorkor

If early malnutrition is not treated, it may develop into marasmus or kwashiorkor or a combination of these two conditions. Marasmus normally occurs in children below one year and is due to eating an insufficient quantity of food.

5

AIDS IN INDIA

AIDS is one of the most dreaded and deadliest diseases of the modern world. It is now a global disease but different human groups differ widely in their understanding of its origin, significance and modes of spread, as well as the meanings they ascribe it, this is another example of a split between disease and illness described in chapter 1.

History

In the spring of 1981, unusual patterns of illnesses were noticed at the center for disease control (CDC) in Atlanta, Georgia, U.S.A, in individuals who were either very young or very old and who had compromised immune systems. Diseases such as *Kapasis Sarcoma* (a type of skin cancer), *toxoplasmosis* (a parasitic disease, usually harmless, often spread by cats and chickens), thrush and herpes began to appear in patients along with severe weight loss and fevers of unknown origin. All these patients were health y ant is the age group of 20-40, which is supposed to be the time of good health and vigour, but on contracting these 'opportunistic' infections were unable to shake them and died as a result. More and more of these cases were reported during the following fall especially in Los Angeles, New York and San Francisco. Surprisingly, it was found that all the early victims were homosexuals, and accordingly this cluster began to be referred to as 'Gay related immune deficiency (GRID)' by many although this was never the official name used at the CDC.

Some early theories tried to determine the causal connection between the life style of the victims and the immune compromise. But, it was discovered in mid-1982 that the syndrome was not confined to the gay community. Intravenous drug users in the same cities began to show the symptoms. This syndrome also began to appear among Haitians and among some females. Next to follow were the Hemophiliacs. In September of 1982, CDC adopted the term 'Acquired Immune Deficiency Syndrome (AIDS). The first cases of AIDS linked to blood transfusions and the first appearance of AIDS in female sexual partners of those in high risk groups were reported by 1982. The communicable retrovirus, which causes AIDS, was discovered and identified in 1984, there by finally eliminating explanations relied exclusively on life styles. With the growing awareness of HIV as the primary cause of the disease, the practice of homosexuality is increasingly stigmatized not on vertical grounds but as a result of moral contagion.

India is one of the largest and most populated countries in the world, with a population of over one billion. Atleast five million of them are currently living with HIV. According to some estimates, India has a greater number of people living with HIV than any other nation in the world (UNAIDS 2006).

HIV emerged much later in India than it did in many other countries, but this has not limited its impact. Infection rates soared throughout the 1990s, and have increased further in recent years. The crisis continues to deepen, as it becomes clearer that the epidemic is affecting *every* sector of Indian society, not just the sex workers and truck drivers that it was originally associated with.

The History of HIV/AIDS in India

At the beginning of 1986, despite over 20,000 reported AIDS cases worldwide, India had no reported cases of HIV or AIDS (Ghosh,1986). There was recognition, though, that this would not be the case for long.

Later in 1986, India's first cases of HIV were diagnosed among sex workers in Chennai, Tamil Nadu. It was noted that contact with foreign visitors had played a role in initial infections among sex workers, and as HIV screening centres were set up across the country there were calls for visitors to be screened for HIV. Gradually, these calls subsided as more attention was paid to ensuring that HIV screening was carried out in blood banks (Kakar and Kakar, 2001).

In 1987 a National AIDS Control Programme was launched to co-ordinate national responses. Its activities covered surveillance, blood screening, and health education (NACO, 2006). By the end of 1987, out of 52,907 who had been tested, around 135 people were found to be HIV positive and 14 had AIDS. Most of these initial cases had occurred through heterosexual sex, but at the end of the 1980s a rapid spread of HIV was observed among injecting drug users in Manipur, Mizoram and Nagaland-three north-eastern states of India bordering Myanmar (Panda, 2002).

At the beginning of the 1990s, as infection rates continued to rise, responses were strengthened. In 1992 the government set up NACO (the National AIDS Control Organisation), to oversee the formulation of policies, prevention work and control programmes relating to HIV and AIDS (Bhupesh, 1992). In the same year, the government launched a Strategic Plan for HIV prevention. This plan established the administrative and technical basis for programme management and also set up State AIDS bodies in 25 states and 7 union territories. It was able to make a number of important improvements in HIV prevention such as improving blood safety.

By this stage, cases of HIV infection had been reported in every state of the country. Throughout the 1990s, it was clear that although individual states and cities had separate epidemics, HIV had spread to the general population. Increasingly, cases of infection were observed among people that had previously been seen as *'low-risk'*, such as housewives and richer members of society.

In 2001, the government adopted the National AIDS Prevention and Control Policy. HIV had now spread extensively throughout the country. A 2004 NACO report revealed that the total number of people living with HIV had risen from 0.2 million in 1990 to 3.86 million in 2000. By 2003, 5.1 million infections had been reported.

Current Estimates

There is disagreement over how many people are currently living with HIV in India. UNAIDS (the United Nations agency that co-ordinates global efforts to fight HIV) estimates that there were 5.7 million people in India living with HIV by the end of 2005, suggesting that India has a higher number of people living with HIV than any other country in the world (UNAIDS,2006). On the other hand, NACO has established an estimate of 5.2 million people, which indicates that there are less infected people in India than in South Africa. Either way, it is clear that the number affected by the epidemic is huge.

By the end of July 2005, the total number of AIDS cases reported to NACO was 111,608. Of this number, 32,567 were women, and 37% were under the age of 30. These figures are not completely accurate reflections of the actual situation though, as large numbers of AIDS cases go unreported.

Overall, around 0.9% of India's population is living with HIV. While this may seem a low rate, India's population is vast, so the actual number of people living with HIV is remarkably high. There are so many people living in India that a mere 0.1% increase in the HIV prevalence would increase the estimated number of people living with HIV by over half a million.

The following states have recorded the highest levels of HIV prevalence at antenatal and sexually transmitted disease (STD) clinics over recent years.

Andhra Pradesh

Andhra Pradesh is a southeran state of the country with a total population of around 76 million, of whom 6 million live in or around the city of Hyderabad. The HIV prevalence at antenatal clinics was around 2% in both 2004 and

2005 higher than in any other state. The vast majority of infections in Andhra Pradesh are believed to result from sexual transmission. HIV prevalence at STD clinics was 22.8% in 2005.

HIV Prevalence in Andhra Pradesh

At the end of 2004, the estimate for HIV positive people in Andhra Pradesh (INDIA) is 5.68 lakhs, which is almost 1/10 of the national figure. Of the 23 districts in AP, 17 districts reported 1% HIV positively, 12 districts reported 2% and above among the pregnant women. 92% of the infected are in the age group of 15-49 years and 88.5% of the infections were through sexual route of transmission. Other modes of transmissions (3.64%) include parents to child transmissions, infected syringes (0.99%), Blood and blood products (0.96%) and others (5.90%).

Conditions for Rapid Growth of HIV in Andhra Pradesh

About one in five men report non-regular sexual partners and the sexually transmitted infections are 7% in both male and female. Another reason is the low rate of condoms use. Large migrant population also contributes to the rapid growth of HIV with increasing trafficking of girls in to sex trade. Existence of strong traditional sexual networks having links to Mumbai, Goa and Pune and vast network of national highways are the other reason.

Goa

Goa is a very small state in the southwest of India, and is best known as a tourist destination. Tourism is so prominent that the number of tourists almost equals the resident population, which is about 1.3 million. The HIV prevalence at antenatal clinics was found to be above 1% in both 2002 and 2004, but was 0.5% in 2003 and 0% in 2005. This variation is likely due to the small number of women tested; the 2005 survey included only two antenatal sites. Prevalence at STD clinics was 14% in 2005, indicating that Goa has a serious epidemic of HIV among sexually active people.

Karnataka

Karnataka-a diverse state in the southwest of India-has a population of around 53 million. In Karnataka the average HIV prevalence at antenatal clinics has exceeded 1% in all recent years. Districts with the highest prevalence tend to be located in and around Bangalore in the southern part of the state, or in northern Karnataka's "devadasi belt". Devadasi women are a group of women who have historically been dedicated to the service of gods. These days, this has evolved into sanctioned prostitution, and as a result many women from this part of the country are supplied to the sex trade in big cities such as Mumbai. The average HIV prevalence among female sex workers in Karnataka was 18% in 2005.

Maharasthra

Mumbai (Bombay) is the capital city of Maharasthra state and is the most populous city in India, with around 20 million inhabitants. Maharastra is a very large state of three hundred thousand square kilometres, with a total population of around 97 million. The HIV prevalence at antenatal clinics in Maharasthra has exceeded 1% in all recent years, and surveys of female sex workers have found rates of infection above 20%. Very high rates are also found among injecting drug users and men who have sex with men.

Tamil Nadu

When surveillance systems in the southern Indian state of Tamil Nadu, home to some 62 million people, showed that HIV infection rates among pregnant women were rising - tripling to 1.25% between 1995 and 1997-the State Government acted decisively. Funding for the Tamil Nadu State AIDS Control Society (TANSACS), which had been set up in 1994, was significantly increased. Along with non-governmental organisations and other partners, TANSACS developed an active AIDS prevention campaign. This included hiring a leading international advertising agency to promote condom use for risky sex in a humorous way, without offending the many people who do not engage in risky behaviour. The campaign also attacked the ignorance and stigma associated with HIV infection.

The HIV prevalence at antenatal clinics in Tamil Nadu was 0.88% in 2002 and 0.5% in 2005, though several districts still have rates above 1%. Prevalence among injecting drug users was 18% in 2005. Tamil Nadu had reported 52,036 AIDS cases to NACO by July 2005, which is by far the highest number of any state.

Manipur

Manipur is a small state of some 2.2 million people in the northeast of India. The nearness of Manipur to Myanmar (Burma), and therefore to the Golden Triangle drug trail, has made it a major transit route for drug smuggling, with drugs easily available. HIV prevalence among injecting drug users is above 20%, and the virus is no longer confined to this group, but has spread further to the female sexual partners of drug users and their children. The HIV prevalence at antenatal clinics in Manipur has exceeded 1% in all recent years.

Mizoram

The small northeastern state of Mizoram has fewer than a million inhabitants. In 1998, an HIV epidemic took off quickly among the state's male injecting drug users, with some drug clinics registering HIV rates of more than 70% among their patients. In recent years the average prevalence among this group has been much lower, at around 5%. HIV prevalence at antenatal clinics has exceeded 1% in most recent years, but was 0.88% in 2005.

Nagaland

Nagaland is another small northeastern state, with a population of two million, where injecting drug use has again been the driving force behind the spread of HIV. In 2005, the HIV prevalence at antenatal clinics was 1.63%, and the rate among injecting drug users was 4.51%.

Who is Affected by HIV and AIDS in India?

People living with HIV in India come from incredibly diverse backgrounds, cultures and lifestyles. The vast majority of infections occur through heterosexual sex, and most of those who become infected would not fall into the category of 'high-risk groups'-although members of such groups, including sex workers, men who have sex with men, truck drivers and migrant workers, do face a proportionately higher risk of infection.

HIV Prevention

Educating people about HIV/AIDS and how it can be prevented is complicated in India, as a number of major languages and hundreds of different dialects are spoken within its population. This means that, although some HIV/AIDS prevention and education can be done at the national level, many of the efforts are best carried out at the state and local level.

Each state has its own AIDS Prevention and Control Society, which carries out local initiatives with guidance from NACO. Under the second stage of the government's National AIDS Control Programme, which finished in March 2006, state AIDS control societies were granted funding for youth campaigns, blood safety checks, and HIV testing among other things. Various public platforms were used to raise awareness of the epidemic-concerts, radio dramas, a voluntary blood donation day and TV spots with a popular Indian film-star. Messages were also conveyed to young people through schools. Teachers and peer educators were trained to teach about the subject, and students were educated through active learning sessions, including debates and role-playing.

The next stage of the National AIDS Control Programme will see US$2.5 billion spent on fighting HIV and AIDS, most of which will be spent on prevention. Aside from the government, this money will come from non-governmental organisations, companies, and international agencies, such as the World Bank and the Bill and Melinda Gates Foundation.

The government has announced that this campaign will place a strong focus on condom promotion. It has already supported the installation of over 11,000 condom vending machines in colleges, road-side restaurants, stations, gas stations and hospitals, and plans to increase this number to 100,000 by the end of 2007. With support from the United States Agency for International Development (USAID), the government has also initiated a campaign called 'Condom Bindas Bol!', which involves advertising, public events and celebrity endorsements. It aims to break the taboo that currently surrounds condom use in India, and to persuade people that they should not be embarrassed to buy them.

In one unique scheme, health activists in West Bengal are attempting to promote condom use through kite flying, which is popular before the state's biggest festival, Durga Puja:

This initiative is an example of how HIV prevention campaigns in India can be tailored to the situations of different states and areas. In doing so, they can make an important impact, particularly in rural areas where information is often lacking. Small-scale campaigns like this are often run or supported by non-governmental organisations, which play a vital role in preventing infections throughout India, particularly among high-risk groups. In some cases, members of these risk groups have formed their own organisations to respond to the epidemic.

Testing

The general consensus among those fighting AIDS worldwide is that HIV testing should be carried out voluntarily, with the consent of the individual concerned. This view has been supported by the Indian government and NACO, who have helped to establish of hundreds of voluntary counselling and testing (VCT) centres in India. By the end of 2005 there were 873 VCT centres in India, compared to just 62 in 1997. These centres tested 225,600 people for HIV during 2005.

Although voluntary testing is officially supported in India, some states have tried to implement policies that would force people to be tested for HIV against their will. In Goa, the state government recently planned to make HIV tests compulsory before marriage, and in Punjab it has been proposed that all people wishing to obtain or retain a driver's license should be tested for HIV. Neither of these plans has come to pass, but they have concerned activists, who argue that HIV testing should never be imposed on people against their wishes.

Unfortunately, cases of people being tested without their consent or knowledge are common in Indian hospitals. In one 2002 study, it was suggested that over 95% of patients listed for surgical procedures are tested against their will, often resulting in their surgery being cancelled. Hospital staff and health professionals, much like the rest of the Indian population, are often unaware of the facts about HIV. This leads to unnecessary fears and, in some cases, causes them to stigmatise HIV positive people and discriminate against them, including testing them without consent.

Treatment for People Living with HIV

HAART–a form of treatment involving antiretroviral drugs (ARVs),which significantly delays the progression from HIV to AIDS–has been available in richer countries since 1996. Unfortunately, as in many poorer countries, access to this treatment is severely limited in India, with only about 95,000 people (less than 15% of those in need) receiving ARVs in India by the end of 2006. Some people manage to access the drugs through private health facilities, which dominate India's healthcare sector, but the vast majority of people cannot afford to buy treatment privately.

While the coverage of treatment remains unacceptably low, improvements are being made. The government has started to expand access to ARVs in a number of areas, and the national number of ARV centres increased from 25 to around 70 in 2005 alone.

There are also plans to improve the provision of nevirapine to pregnant mothers with HIV, which can significantly reduce the risk that they will pass infection on to their child. It has been reported that, even where treatment to prevent mother-to-child-transmission is available, some women do not request it because of the stigma surrounding HIV.

The large scale of India's epidemic, the diversity of its spread, and the country's lack of finances and resources all present barriers to India's programme. Ironically, India is a major provider of cheap generic copies of ARVs to countries all over the world.

Stigma and Discrimination in India

In India, as elsewhere, AIDS is often seen as *"someone else's problem"*–as something that effects people living on the margins of society, whose lifestyles are considered immoral. Even as it moves into the general population, the HIV epidemic is misunderstood and stigmatised among the Indian public. People living with HIV have faced violent attacks; been rejected by families, spouses and communities; been refused medical treatment; and even, in some reported cases, denied the last rites before they die.

As well as adding to the suffering of people living with HIV, this discrimination is hindering efforts to prevent new infections. While such strong reactions to HIV and AIDS exist, it is difficult to educate people about how they can avoid infection. AIDS outreach workers and peer-educators have reported harassment, and in schools, teachers sometimes face negative reactions from the parents of children that they teach about AIDS:

Discrimination is also alarmingly common in the health care sector. Negative attitudes from health care staff have generated anxiety and fear among many people living with HIV and AIDS. As a result, many keep their status secret. It is not surprising that among a majority of HIV positive people, AIDS-related fear and anxiety, and at times denial of their HIV status, can be traced to traumatic experiences in health care settings.

A 2006 study found that 25% of people living with HIV in India had been refused medical treatment on the basis of their HIV-positive status. It also found strong evidence of stigma in the workplace, with 74% of employees not disclosing their status to their employees for fear of discrimination. Of the 26% who did disclose their status, 10% reported having faced prejudice as a result (UNDP, 2006),. People in marginalized groups-female sex workers, hijras (transgender) and gay men-are often stigmatised not only because of their HIV status, but also because they belong to socially excluded groups.

The Future of HIV and AIDS in India

Various groups have made predictions about the effect that AIDS will have on India in the future, and there has been a lot of dispute about the accuracy of these estimates. For instance, a 2002 report by the CIA's National Intelligence Council predicted 20 million to 25 million AIDS cases in India by 2010-more than any other country in the world. Yet the government has claimed that these figures are "completely inaccurate", and has accused those who cite them of "spreading panic". The government has also disputed predictions that India's epidemic is "on an African trajectory", although it claims to acknowledge the seriousness of the crisis.

Ruben del Prado, deputy UNAIDS country coordinator for India, has predicted that "there is going to be a reversal of the epidemic by 2008 and 2009".This does not correlate with other UN-related estimates, however, which have suggested that:

- India's adult HIV prevalence will peak at 1.9% in 2019.
- The number of AIDS deaths in India (which was estimated at 2.7 million for the period 1980-2000) will rise to 12.3 million during 2000-15, and to 49.5 million during 2015-50.
- Economic growth in India will slow by almost a percentage point per year as a result of AIDS by 2019.

Today AIDS is the third biggest killer in the world. According to UNAIDS, at the end of 2004, 42 million people are living with HIV/AIDS and there were 5.13 million new infections and 3.1 million deaths occurred. If we look at the global scenario, every day 14,000 new infections occur. Of these 2,000 infections were among those below 14 years age (primarily through vertical transmission). Out of the 12,000 infections occurring in the age groups of 15 years and above, 50% of infections (i.e., 6000) occur in the age group of 15-24 years placing the young people in the center of the epidemic.

HIV estimates for India grew enormously since 1990. In 1990 it was 0.2 million and by 1994 it went up to 1.7 million. In 1998 it was 3.5 million and by 2000 it went up to 3.86 million. For 2001 it was 3.97 million while it was 4.58 million in 2002 and in 2003 it reached 5.1 million. Nearly 80% of people with HIV/AIDS in South Asia are in India and the reasons for such a high prevalence could be traced to a host of socio-economic, cultural and biological factors. Andhra Pradesh is one of the top three states in India in registering highest number of HIV/ AIDS cases only next to Maharastra and Tamil Nadu.

Whatever the exact figures turn out to be, it is clear that HIV and AIDS will have a devastating effect on India in the future, and that as much as possible needs to be done to minimise this impact.

The Role of Anthropology

Along side the international effort towards a more comprehensive scientific view of the epidemic and general availability of medical treatment, information/education/ communication (IEC) is a key instrument in the efficient prevention and support to infected and sick people in the perspective of sustainable human development. In order to give it full significance and long-term effects, it has to be elaborated and developed within the context of the cultural approach. In other words, the validity of ICE is and will be tested through the response of population that will result either in continuity or change in their ways of thinking, value systems and styles of life in relation to the epidemic. Who could be better than an Anthropologist to handle such a situation, as the key concept in anthropology is 'Culture'. An Anthropologist's participant observation method makes him eventually a member of the community while doing field work and evidently he would be able to convincingly talk to people in changing their life styles, ways of thinking and value systems, with the ultimate goal to define conditions for their sensitization and mobilization in prevention and care. In addition, valuable IEC activity can work effectively with the collaboration of an Anthropologist with analyzing in–depth specific characters of target audiences, identifications and segmentation of the various "risk group" in their cultural relations with socio-economic development and general society. The culture approach means that any given population's culture reference and resources, such as way of life, value system, traditions and beliefs and the fundamental human rights, will be considered as key references in building a framework for strategies and project planning. These key references will also serve as the resources and basics for building a relevant response and sustainable action in prevention and care as well as in impact reduction. This becomes an indispensable condition to achieve in-depth and long-term changes in people's behaviour and to give full consistency to medical and sanitary strategies. Thus the cultural approach to AIDS and drug abuse problem as well is the best-suited method and Anthropologists are well equipped to handle the situation. Chapter VII portrays the role of Anthropologists in programme design and successful implementation.

6

DRINKING WATER AND DISEASES

Water is the prime-sustaining element for life on earth. The linkage between safe drinking water and health and productivity of human beings is well established. Hence the manner of utilization of water and its disposal have a close bearing on the morbidity and mortality of human beings. Safe drinking water could make a tremendous impact on the quality of life in our villages, because non-availability of safe drinking water has direct impact on the working conditions and health of the people and their productive capacity. It has been noticed that the problem of supply of potable drinking water to different tribal village is very complex and challenging. This chapter presents the quality of drinking water in four tribal villages, two from the plains and two from hill top, undertaken in two case studies.

The prevalence of water borne diseases is very high among the tribals. This high prevalence is usually due to certain behavioural practices and the quality of drinking water. Bore well water is usually considered safe as compared to river or open well water. Drinking water samples of bore wells from Gangannadoravalasa and Reddavalasa tribal villages of Vizianagram District in Andhra Pradesh were analyzed and Microbiological analysis of these waters samples showed high coliforms with high total plate counts. These results indicate high contamination of the water with pathogenic micro-organisms, thereby causing frequent fevers, diarrhea, dysentery and gastroenteritis.

It is too well known that almost all human settlements lie nearby a water point. In the agency area, each tribal settlement is usually situated near a hill stream (*gedda)* or spring (*oota neeru).* The tribal people in this area refer to any type of water resource as *ganga* (sacred water) and it has religious significance. In an earlier study (Elizabeth, *et.al.* 2000) it was found that the river and spring waters in some tribal areas are highly contaminated. In order to mitigate the drinking water problem the State Government has provided bore wells in many tribal villages in this region.

According to the 1991 census, Vizianagaram District in Andhra Pradesh has a tribal population of 1,52,335 which is 7.8% of the total district population. The predominant tribes of the district are: Jatapus, Savaras, Konda doras, Mooka doras, Manne doras and Gadabas. Gangannadoravalasa, a plains village and Reddavalasa , a hill top village, are two tribal villages of Vizianagram District inhabited by Konda dora and Jatapu/savara tribals respectively. Both the villages come under Pachipenta Primary Health Centre.

Material and Method

Water samples were collected from the bore wells of Gangannadoravalasa and Reddavalasa villages in sterile containers and the samples were stored at 4°C at least until the microbiological analysis was completed. The MPN (Most Probable Number), test is related to coliform group of bacteria. *Escherichia coli* and *Enterobacter aerogenes* belong to this group, which are usually found in the normal flora of human intestines. Each day humans as well as animals excrete large number of *E.Coli* through faeces. Therefore, the presence of *E. Coli* in drinking water is generally considered as an indicator of fecal contamination. However, most of the *E. Coli* strains are non-pathogenic except a few toxigenic strains. But the problem shoots up with the contamination by other pathogenic microorganisms simultaneously excreted, leading to several water borne diseases such as typhoid, para-typhoid, other fevers, cholera, diarrhea, bacillary dysentery, amoebic dysentery, hepatitis, and polio. MPN test, which includes presumptive, confirmatory and completed tests, therefore, is performed to estimate the number of coliforms in the water samples.

The total plate count test was done in order to determine the magnitude of bacterial pollution in the sample. This test involves the serial dilution of the sample. Standard aliquots of various dilutions were placed on nutrient agar plates and incubated at 37^{0}C for 18-24 hrs. The plate which showed colony-forming units (cfu) between 30-300 is considered for making total plate counts as that number was statistically significant (Pelczar *et. al.* 1987).

The physical parameters such as p^H, salinity conductivity and turbidity were determined using various standard meters. For chemical analysis of the water, standard methods (APHA, 1985, Suess1982) were followed. Fluoride ions were estimated by using fluoride meter (EWCOOCL 132 model). Spectrophotometric (Systranics 2 V-VIS) technique was used to measure the concentrations of Iron, Phosphates, Nitrates, and Sulphates. The other parameters were estimated by standard volumetric procedures. All concentrations for chemical parameters were expressed in mg/L.

Results and Discussion

The results were given in Table 1. The permissible limit for coliform count is 0-1/100 ml. In this present study, the bore waters from Gangannadora Valasa and Redda Valasa showed 49 and 45 coliforms/100 ml respectively, as determined by MPN Method, clearly indicating that these waters were non-potable due to microbes. The total plate count of the two water samples tested in the present study were very high, that is 1.0 x 10^4 Cfu/ ml 2.0x10^3 cfu/ml from Gangannadora Valasa and Redda valasa villages respectively suggesting that the waters are not potable. These results correlate well with our current data collected from Pachipenta Primary Health Centre (unpublished) where there was high incidence of fevers, diarrhea, dysentery, and gastroenteritis. The poor health status of these tribals is also due to the regular consumption of highly pathogen-contaminated waters.

Table 1
Analysis of Drinking Water in Two Tribal Villages of Vizianagaram District

Parameters Tested	*Bore water from Ganagannadora Valasa Village*	*Bore water form Reddavalasa Village*	*Drinking water Standards of ICMR & WHO*
Microbiological Parameters			
MPN Test	49 coliforms/ 100 ml sample	49 coliforms/ 100 ml sample	0-1 coliform count
Total plate count	1.0 x 10^4 cfu/ml	2.0 x 10^2 cfu/ ml	100 cfu. Ml
Physico-chemical Parameters			
p^H	7.9	7.25	6.5-8.5
Turbidity	.80 NTU	0.30 NTU	5.0 NTU
Salinity	0.0%	0.0%	0.0-0.5 %
Conductivity	1.3 m Mhos	0.9m Mhos	2.5m Mhos
Chemical Parameters			
Total Solids (TS)	800 mg/L	800 mg/L	500mg-1000mg
Total dissolved solids (TDS)	400 mg/L	600 mg/L	500- 1500mg/L
Total suspended solids (TSS)	400 mg/L	200 mg/L	500 mg/L
Total Hardness mg/L.	296 mg/L	256 mg/L	75 mg/L-200
Calcium hardness	113 mg/ L	96 mg/L	50-100 mg/ L
Magnesium hardness	184 mg/L	160 mg/L	
Chlorides	127.7 mg/L	87.0 mg/L	250 mg/L
Flurides	1.59ppm/L	0.401 ppm/L	1.2ppm/L
Nitrates	3.08 mg / L	4.0 mg / L	45 mg/L
Sulphates	200mg/L	700mg/L	250mg/L
Phosphates	2.0mg/L	6.0mg/L	250 mg/L
Iron	054mg/L	03 mg/L	0.2mg/L

Regarding the physico-chemical properties of the drinking water, the p^H is very important parameter upon which all biochemical reactions are dependent. In the present study the

p^H, turbidity, salinity, and conduciivity of the two water samples were within the permissible limits indicating that the waters are potable with respect to physical factors. The total solids of these bore well waters have exceeded the lower limit but not the upper limit, therefore potable. The total dissolved solids (TDS) in bore well water of Reddavalasa Village was 600mg/L which has exceeded the lower limit of TDS for drinking water sample, therefore chemically non potable as it may posses dissolved carcinogenic chemicals.

The total hardness in Gangannadora Valasa bore well waters was 296 mg/L and that of Redda Valasa was 256/L. They have exceeded the upper permissible limit for total hardness. As the hardness of water causes formation of stones in the kidneys and others impairments in human physiology, these waters are non-potable.

The calcium hardness in bore waters of Gangannadora Valasa was higher, i.e. 112 mg/L. than the permissible limit, suggesting that consumption of such waters may cause stone formation in kidneys. In the present investigation, the fluoride content in the bore waters of Gangannadora valasa is very high, i.e. 1.54 ppm/L than the normal permissible limit which is 1.22-1.5 ppm/L (WHO, 1971). High fluoride concentration causes flourosis in adults and fluoride concentration below the lower limit causes dental carries in children. It was also reported that high fluoride content in drinking water causes biochemical effects such as high blood sugar levels, reduced hormonal levels and reduced secondary sexual characters (Deshkar *et.al.* 1998).

In the present study the iron content in bore waters of Gangannadora Valasa was very high, i.e. 0.5 mg/L, whereas that of Reddavalasa was 0.3 mg/L, which exceeded the normal limit indicating that the waters were non-potable. High iron content in the water also promotes the growth of microbes and for that reason high bacterial counts were noticed in these samples. Other chemical parameters such as nitrates, sulphates, and phosphates of the water samples were tested and they were found to be within the permissible limits.

Conclusion

These results clearly indicate that the bore well waters of Gangannadora Valasa and Redda Valasa were highly contaminated with microbes and the high prevalence of morbidities among the tribals of these two villages obviously could be related to the regular consumption of these contaminated waters. Although the tribals usually draw their drinking water from the bore wells, their practice of open defecation or dumping human and animal excreta near the bore wells might have caused the bacteria to leach and pollute the ground water.

The hardness, fluorides, and iron content in the waters of Gangannadora Valasa were very high when compared to those of Redda Valasa Village suggesting that the Redda Valasa water is more potable than that of Gangannadora Valasa Village. The chemical toxicity of water may also cause poor health of these villagers.

As the physico-Chemical properties cannot be changed easily, it is advisable for the tribals to boil and cool the water before consumption. Boiling water helps kill the microbes and cooling helps settling of minerals like, calcium, magnesium etc., and it also removes some of the hardness.

Another study of similar nature was undertaken to confirm the results of the earlier study. The microbiological and physic-chemical parameters of drinking water samples from two villages of Vizianagarm District were monitored. The microbiological analysis of Janjavathi river water showed very high faecal coliform counts and large number of colony forming units (cfu) i.e., 540/100ml and 2.18×10^8/ml as determined by MPN test and standard total plate count methods respectively. Borewell water from Sominaiduvalasa village showed 1600 coliforms per 100ml sample and 4.3×10^9 cfu/ml, suggesting that these waters are highly polluted with microbial pathogens and therefore, non-potable. Physico-chemical parameters such as pH, conductivity, Total Solids (TS), Total Dissolved Solids (TDS), total hardness, Calcium hardness, Magnesium hardness, chlorides, fluorides, sulphates and Iron were beyond the permissible limits in borewell water indicating that this water is non-potable.

High incidence of water borne diseases viz., gastroenteritis, amoebiasis, bacillary dysentery and occasional cholera among the tribals could be partly due to their unhygienic water which possess higher amounts of minerals and other pathogenic microorganisms than the permissible limits. As the quality of drinking water available in Vizianagaram sub-plan area has not been scientifically established so far, it is conceived in this study to collect drinking water samples from various sources like springs, rivers, bore wells and conduct microbiological, physico-chemical tests.

Water samples were collected from Janjavathi River in Banjukuppa village, with a total population of 240, inhabitated by Jatapu and Savara tribes, and borewell water from Sominaiduvalasa village, with a total population of 630, inhabited by Jatapu and Konda Dora tribes. Several other tribal villages use Janjavathi river water as a source of drinking water. These two villages are situated in Komarada Mandal and come under Komarada and K.R.B. Puram P.H.Cs respectively. The results of various parameters tested were compared with standard permissible limits.

Material and Methods

The water samples were collected in sterile containers and immediately stored in the refrigerator until the microbiological analysis was completed. For microbiological analysis, two methods employed were MPN (Most Probable Number) and standard total plate count method. MPN test was performed in order to detect Escherichia coli, the indicator organism, and its presence in water samples may be scored as positive for faecal contamination of drinking water. The total plate count reveals the magnitude of bacterial contamination of the sample. Total plate count was done using serial dilutions of water samples. The physical parameters of water samples such as pH, salinity, turbidity, and conductivity were determined, using specific meters. The chemical parameters such as the total solids, total dissolved solids, total suspended solids, total hardness, calcium hardness, magnesium hardness, chlorides, fluorides, nitrates, sulphates, phosphates and iron were analysed in the laboratory as per the standard methods (APHA, 1985; SUESS, 1982). Various types of hardness and chlorides were estimated using volumetric analysis. The fluorides were estimated by using fluoride meter (Elico-CL 352 model). The nitrates, phosphates, sulphates and iron were estimated by Spectrophotometric methods (systronics). All the concentrations were expressed in mg/L of water samples.

Results and Discussion

The results of microbiological and physico-chemical parameters of janjavathi river water from Banjukuppa Village and bore waters from Sominaidu valasa are given in Table 2. The permissible limit for Coliform bacteria in drinking water sample is 1/100 ml of sample. But in the present study the coliform count is very high, i.e., 540 coliforms/100ml sample and 1600 coliforms/100ml in Janjavathi river and bore waters respectively, suggesting that these waters are highly contaminated with faecal matter and are non-potable. The results of the present study correlate well with the data collected from KRB Puram Primary Health Center which showed high incidence of fevers, diarrhea, dysentery and gastroenteritis (unpublished data). The MPN test is used to detect the presence of coliform bacteria, especially *Echerichia coli,* the indicator organism in drinking water. *E. coli* is the normal inhabitant of human and animal intestines. Every day millions of *E. coli* are excreted out through human and animal faeces. Presence of coliforms in drinking water is a strong indication for the presence of various pathogenic microorganisms which have been excreted out simultaneously with *coliforms.* These microbial pathogens may be *Salmonella typhi,* the causative agent of typhoid, *S. paratyph,* the causative agent of paratyphoid, *Vibrio cholerae,* the causative agent of cholera, *Shigella dysenteriae,* the causative agent of bacillary dysentery, *Entamoeba histolytica* of amebiasis, *Yersinia enterocolitica, Y. pseudotuberculosis, E. coli* (toxigenic and entero-invasive strains) that cause diarrhea and gastroenteritis. The viral waterborne diseases may be due to the presence of pathogenic virus in waters such as *Hepatitis-A,* the causative agent of jaundice and *Polio myelitis* Virus which cause polio.

In the present investigation the standard total plate count was 2.1×10^8 and 4.3×10^9 cfu/ml in Janjavathi river water and bore waters respectively. These results exceeded the permissible limit which should be only <100cfu/1ml. These results suggest high incidence of fevers, diarrhea, dysentery and gastroenteritis among the tribals of Vizianagaram District.

Table 2
Microbiological and Physico-chemical Parameters of Drinking Water Samples from Two Tribal Villages of Vizianagaram District

Parameters Tested	*Janjavathi river water from Banjukuppa village*	*Borewell water from Sominaiduvalasa village*	*Permissible Limits*
Microbiological Parameters			
MPN Test	540 Coliforms/ 100ml sample	1600 Coliforms/ 100ml sample	1 coliform/ 100ml sample
Total Plate count	2.1×10^8 cfu/ 1ml sample	4.3×10^9 cfu/ 1ml sample	<100cfu/1ml sample
Physical Parameters			
pH	8.7	7.78	6.5-8.5
Turbidity	0.8 NTU	NTU	5.0 NTU
Salinity	0.01%	0.0%	0.0%
Conductivity	0.6 mMhos	3.4 mMhos	<2.5mMhos
Chemical Parameters			
Total Solids (TS)	400mg/L	2200 mg/L	500-1000 mg/L
Total Dissolved Solids (TDS)	300 mg/L	2200 mg/L	500-1000 mg/L
Total Suspended Solids (TDS)	100 mg/L	0.0mg/L	500 mg/L
Total Hardness	156/L	848 mg/L	75-200 mg/L
Calcium Hardness	96 mg/L	112mg/L	50-100 mg/L
Magnesium Hardness	60 mg/L	736 mg/L	50-100 mg/L
Chlorides	464 mg/L	1341 mg/L	250 mg/L
Fluorides	0.504 ppm/L	1.22 ppm/L	1.2-1.5 ppm/L
Nitrates	3.5 mg/L	8.8mg/L	45 mg/L
Sulphates	200 mg/L	500 mg/L	250 mg/L
Phosphates	2.0ug/L	2.5ug/L	250 mg/L
Iron	0.4 mg/L	0.5 mg/L	0.2 mg/L

The pH of water is one of the important physical factors as all biochemical reactions occur at specific pH and are dependent on pH. Usually water sample with a pH of 7 is considered the best but the permissible limit ranges between 6.5-8.5 (ICMR, 1975). In the present study the Janjavathi river water has a pH of 8.71, which was beyond the permissible range where as the bore well water has a pH of 7.78. In the microbiological perspective, the river water pH favours the growth of Vibrio species, which ultimately cause diarrhea. The salinity of these waters was 0.0% which was within the limits, suggesting that the waters do not taste saltish and are therefore potable.

The conductivity of water is an important parameter, which determines the drinking water quality and also water used for agricultural purposes. The permissible limit of conductivity for drinking water is <2.5 mMhos. In the present study the conductivity of bore water was 3.4 mMhos which exceeded the normal limit suggesting high concentration of charged ions in the water which eventually makes the water non-potable. The turbidity of water is imported by the total suspended solid particles. The permissible limit for drinking water sample is 5.0 NTU (Nephelo Turbidity Units). In the present investigation the turbidity of tested waters is within the desirable limit suggesting that there was less amount of suspended particles in the waters. The total solids of drinking water should not exceed 500mg/L which may be due to the presence of total suspended solids or total dissolved solids or both. In the present study the total solids of river water was within the limits (400mg/L) but the bore water showed very high value of 2200 mg/L indicating that the bore water was non-potable. The permissible limit of TDS is 500mg/L, but should never exceed the maximum permissible limit of 1500mg/L (ICMR, 19750). In the present investigation the TDS of bore waters from Sominaiduvalasa village is very high i.e., 2200mg/L indicating high degree of dissolved toxic chemicals, which were non-filterable and may be carcinogenic. The high TDS results in bad taste, strain on kidney, impact on digestion, blood pressure and other metabolic disturbances. The total suspended solids of river water was 100mg/L, where as that of bore water was

0.0mg/L. The river water showed little turbidity i.e., 0.08 NTU but the bore waters showed 0.0 NTU as it did not contain any suspended solids but possessed only the dissolved solids.

The total hardness of potable water should not exceed the permissible limit of 200 mg/L (ICMR, 1975) otherwise it may lead to stone formation in kidneys. In the present study bore well water has very high content of total hardness i.e., 848mg/L. The desirable limit for Calcium hardness in drinking water ranges between 75-200 mg/L, whereas for Magnesium it is 50-100 mg/L (ICMR, 1975). Calcium and Magnesium sulphates beyond the permissible limit will act as purgatives and may lead to respiratory diseases (Maiti, 1982). In this study the Magnesium hardness of bore water is very high (736mg/L). The chloride content of potable water should not exceed the maximum permissible limit of 250 mg/L. But, in the present study the river and bore well waters showed high content of chlorides i.e., 464 mg/L and 134 mg/L respectively indicating that there may be sewage or faecal contamination in the river water or the presence of Magnesium chloride rock formation below the ground level, indicating that the water is non-potable. The Sulphates of bore water was 500 mg/L, exceeding the normal limit, indicates that the water may act as purgative.

The Fluoride content of drinking water should not exceed the maximum permissible limit of 1.5 mg/L (WHO, 1971) due to which severe bone diseases called fluorosis may occur. If the fluoride content is <0.2 mg/L, it may lead to dental carries in children. In the present study the bore waters are almost near the maximum permissible limit suggesting that the water is non-potable. Recently it has been reported that fluorides in the fluorosis patients have adversely affected various hormonal levels and the development of secondary sexual characters (Deshkar, *et al.*, 1998). The nitrates in drinking water should not exceed the maximum limit of 45 mg/L which when exceeds may lead to blue babies (NRC, 1972) and anemia in humans. This study showed that the nitrate content was within the limits. The phosphate content of the samples tested were within the limits. The iron content of drinking water should not exceed 0.3 mg/L but in the present study the water samples tested exceeded the normal limit., i.e., 0.4 mg/L and 0.5 mg/L in river and bore waters respectively, suggesting that these waters taste bad and are non-potable.

Conclusion

The results presented in the two case studies clearly indicate that both the river and the bore-well waters are highly polluted with pathogenic microorganisms, through fecal contamination. Regarding the high counts in bore well water, there may be open defaecation or dumping yards near the bore well and the coliforms might have leached into the ground waters causing microbiological pollution which ultimately leads to various water borne diseases. The total hardness, Magnesium hardness, Chlorides, total dissolved solids and iron content are very high in bore waters than the river water. Therefore, the people should drink boiled water which may eliminate microbiological and chemical pollution of water to some extent. But the toxic effects caused by heat stable toxins of pathogens cannot be removed by boiling the water.

7

THE SHAMAN

Explanations in magico-religious domain are divinatory in nature unlike scientific explanations in all other domains. As magico-religious personnel mediate with supernatural, a certain body of ceremonial/ritual knowledge evolved over a period of time everywhere. Many parts of the world are inhabited by a bewildering variety of tribal people. Magico-religious personnel in this region viz., the priests, magicians, shaman or the medicine men are very popular among these tribal populations and literature on shamanism/medicine-man is available aplenty. The following is an account of shaman among certain tribes of Asia Pacific region, where the role of the shaman is very important in the lives of the tribals, and comparisons are made with the shaman of other areas in South India.

The Shaman

Shamanism basically refers to the religious phenomenon of Siberia and Central Asia. The word 'Shamanism comes through Russian, from Tungusic, 'saman'. The derivation of this word from pali 'samana' (Sanskrit sramana) through the Chinese shamen (a mere transcription of the Pali word), which was accepted by majority of the ninteenth century Orientalists was nevertheless questioned and rejected by Schott, Nemeth and Laufer. The corresponding words in other languages are, 'ojuna'

(Yakut), 'bugal', 'boga' and 'udagan' (Mangolian), 'kam' (Turko-Tatar), 'samana' (Pali). The Siberian Shaman's ec-static experience expresses the meaning of the word 'Shamanism' as 'the technique of ecstasy' (Eliade, 1974:4). In popular literature, the terms, 'shaman', 'medicine-man', 'sorcerer', and 'magician' are interchangeably used.

The Office

The chief methods of recruiting shamans in Central and North-east Asia are, 1. hereditary transmission of the shaman's profession (e.g., samoyed, ostyak, votyak) and 2. Spontaneous vocation ('call' or 'vocation'). There are also cases of individuals who became shamans of their own free will (Altaians), or by the will of the clan as in case of Tungus (Eliade, 1974: 13).

South-east Asian and Oceanic Shamanism

The Semang, the Sakai, and the Jakun

The medicine man of the Semang is called Hala or halak, a term also employed by the Sakai. If some one falls ill, the hala (Sakai) or the poyang (Jakun: variant of the Malayan term pawang) and his assistant retire to a leaf hut and begin singing to invoke the cenoi, 'the nephews of God'. After some time the voices of the cenoi themselves rise from the hut; the hala and his assistant sing and speak in an unknown language, which when they leave the hut, they profess to have forgotten. Actually, the cenoi have sung through their mouths. The descent of these luminous spirits is manifested by hut shaking. It is they who reveal the cause of the illness and indicate the treatment; and it is on this occasion that the hala is supposed to go into trance (Evans, 1923: 115). During his seance the hala holds threads made from palm leaves or very fine cords. These threads and cords reach the celestial god who dwells above the seven levels of the sky. As long as the seance continues, the hala is directly connected with the celestial god by these threads or cords, which the god sends down and, after the ceremony, draws back to himself. Finally, an essential element in the cure is quartz crystals. These crystals can be directly obtained from the cenoi or they can be prepared; cenoi are believed to live in these magical stones and to be at hala's orders. The healer is said to see sickness in these crystals; that is the cenoi inside them show him the cause of the sickness and the treatment for it. But in these crystals the hala himself can see a tiger approaching the camp. The hala himself can turn into a tiger just like the Malayan shamans and shamanesses indicating Malayan influence, ft is to be noted here that the mythical Tiger Ancestor is regarded throughout South-east Asia as the initiatory master; it is he who takes the neophytes to the jungle to initiate them (in reality to 'kill' and 'revive' them). In other words the tiger forms part of an extremely archaic religious complex.

Malaya

What is called Malayan shamanism has as its distinctive characteristics the evocation of the tiger spirit and obtaining the condition of lupa. It is a state of unconsciousness into which the shaman falls and during which the spirits descend on him, possess him, and answer questions put by the audience. Whether the case is one of individual cure or a ceremony of collective defense against epidemics, the Malayan seance usually includes the evocation of the tiger, for the purpose of summoning and securing the incarnation of the mythical ancestor, the first Great Shaman. This is because the role of mythical ancestor and, hence, of initiatory master, is given to the tiger throughout this area (Skeat, 1900:436). The magical dances culminate in lupa, and the healer makes use of the trance to ask questions and discover the causes of the illness and treatment for it.

Sumatra

Religious ideas are dominated in Sumatra by the concept of the soul (tone); it enters and leaves the body through the fontanel. Death is, in reality, the abduction of the soul by a spirit (begu); if the deceased is a young man, a woman begu has laken him for her husband, and vice versa. The dead and the spirits speak through mediums. The shaman is called 'sibaso', and the priest is called 'datu'. Although they differ in structure and religious vocation, they pursue the same end—defending the soul against being abducted by demons, ensuring the integrity of the human person. The sibaso seance takes place in the night; the shaman drums and dances around the fire to invoke the spirits. Each spirit has its particular melody and even its special colour, and the sibaso wears a costume of several colours if he wishes to invoke several spirits. Their presence is manifested by words uttered by the sibaso in secret language, the 'language of the spirits', which must be interpreted. The dialogue concerns the causes of the illness and the means of curing it; the begu promises that it will perform a cure if the patient will offer certain sacrifices (Loeb, 1935: 81).

Borneo and Celebes

Among the Dyak of the interior there are two kinds of magician-healers: daya beruri, usually men, whose field is healing, and barich, commonly recruited among women, specialists in the 'treatment' of paddy harvests. Illness is interpreted either as the presence of an evil spirit in the body or as the absence of the soul. Shamans of both classes have ecstatic power to see the human soul or the soul of the harvest, even if these have fled to great distances. They then pursue the fugitive souls, capture them (in the form of a hair), and restore them to their place in the body (or the crops). When the illness is caused by an evil spirit, the seance is reduced to an expulsion ceremony (Roth, 1896: 259-63). Miles observes that in most pagan communities. Seances take place nearly every week when a hundred or more spirits may descend during a sincle ceremony. Amongst them some are renowned for the ability to cure certain ailments, some give a guarantee of success in farming and gardening, whereas some bring safety to hunting expeditions. Spirits performing services expect appropriate remuneration, resulting in the formation of a subsequent seance held specifically in the benefactor's honour. Thus one ceremony brings forth to another (1966: 3).

Melanesia

In general, three types of culture are distinguishable in Melanesia, each disseminated by one of the three ethnic groups that would seem to have colonized (or merely passed through) the area: the aboriginal Papuans, the white-skinned conquerors who brought agriculture, megaliths, and other forms of civilization and then moved on to Polynesia, and the black-skinned Melanesians, the last to reach the islands (Riesenfed, 1950: 655-680). The white-skinned immigrants disseminated a very rich mythology, centered about a culture hero (Qat, Ambat) who has direct relations with the sky, whether by marrying a celestial fairy, whom, after the precaution to steal and hide her wings, he pursues to the sky by climbing a tree, a vine or a chain arrows, or because he himself a native of the celestial region. The myths of Qat correspond to the Polynesian myths of Tagarao and maui, whose relations with the sky and celestial beings are well known.

In Melanesia we observe, together with techniques of magical cure whose archaism seems beyond doubt, the absence of a properly shamanic tradition and initiation. The disappearance of shamanic initiation could be attributed to the large role played by secret societies based on initiations. The essential function of the Melanesian medicine men is thus restricted to healing and divination. Certain other specifically shamanic powers (magical flight) remain the almost exclusive prerogative of black magicians. Indeed, what is generally called shamanism is no where so divided up among a multitude of magico-religious groups as it is in Oceania, and especially in Melanesia, where we can distinguish priests, medicine men, sorcerers, diviners, the 'processed' etc. A number of motifs that in one way or another form part of the shamanic ideology survive only in myths or funerary beliefs. Seligman (1910: 158,273) reported a belief among them that the deceased, on reaching the land of the dead, is subjected by its guardian to the mutilation of ear piercing. Now, this operation is distinctive of shamanic initiations.

In Dobu, one of the islands to the east of New Guinea, illness is brought on either by magic or by the spirits of the dead. The medicine man is summoned to discover the cause of the illness by gazing into crystals or water. In his crystal the healer sees the person, living or dead, who has brought on the illness. The living author of the charm is paid to cease his hostility, or offerings are made to the dead man who proves to be the cause of illness (Fortune, 1932: 154). In the Banks Islands the illness is expelled by massages or by suction; the shaman then shows the patient a bit of bone or wood or a leaf, and makes him drink water in which magical stones have been placed (Codrington, 1981:194). The same technique is found in Fiji.

Polynesia

Matters are further complicated in Polynesia as there are several classes of specialists in the sacred, all of them having more or less direct relations with the gods and spirits. Broadly speaking, we find three great categories of religious functionaries: the divine chiefs (ariki), the prophets (tula), and the priests (tohunga), but to these we must add healers, sorcerers, necromancers, and the spontaneously 'possessed', all of whom, employ more or less the same technique: entry into contact with the gods or spirits, inspiration or possession by them. Handy (1923) opines that some of the religious ideologies and techniques have been influenced by Asian ideas.

In Polynesia, sickness is attributed to an object introduced into the body by a god or a spirit, or to possession. And treatment consists in extracting the magical object or expelling the spirit. But, in Polynesia healing is not the exclusive prerogative of the medicine man, as it is in Australia and elsewhere; the extreme frequency of possession by gods and spirits has made it possible for healers to proliferate. Priests, inspired persons, medicine men, sorcerers, all can undertake magical cures.

The Indian Tribes

The magicians of the Oraons in Bengal seeks the patients strayed souls through the mountains and rivers and on into the land of the dead (Clements, 1932:197) exactly like the Altaic and Siberian shamans. Elwin's (1947,1949,1955) studies on the Savaras (also spelled as saora) of Orissa throw light on the Indian shamans and shamanesses. It is interesting to note astonishing similarities between them and Siberian shamans especially with reference to the 'initiatory marriages'. "There are, however two differences: (1) since the Savara have both shamans and shamanesses—and sometimes the latter even outnumber the former-both sexes enter into these marriages with an other world being; (2) where as the 'celestial wives' of the Siberian shamans live in the heavens or, in some cases' in the bush, the spiritual spouses of the Savara all inhabit the underworld, the kingdom of shades" (Eliade, 1974: 421).

The Savara shamanic seance consists in the shaman being possessed by the spirit of the tutelary or by the god, whichever is invoked, who speaks through his voice at great length. It is the spirit that takes possession of the shaman or shamaness that reveals the cause of the illness and tells them what action is to be taken (usually a sacrifice or offerings). "Shamanism through possession is also known in other parts of India" (p. 424).

The 'spirit marriage' of the Savara shamans appears to be a unique phenomenon aboriginal India; In any case it is not of Kolarian origin. Rahmann (1959:681-760:722-754) gives the following observations:

1. "Supernatural" election of the future shaman is indispensable among the savara, the Bondo, the Birhor, and the Baiga. Among the Baiga, the Khond and the Bondo "supernatural" election is necessary even if the shaman's office is hereditary. Among the Juang, the Birhor, the Oroan, and the Muria the "elect" usually exhibit psychic traits characteristic of shamanism. (Rahmann 1959: 730)
2. Systematic instruction of future shamans is obligatory in a considerable number of tribes (Santal, Munda, Savara, Baiga, Oroan, Bhil etc.). An initiation ceremony is clearly documented among the Santal, the Munda, the Baiga, the Oroan and the Bhil.
3. Shamans have personal tutelary spirits among the Santal, the Savara, the Korwa, the Birhor, the Bhuiya, the Baiga, the Oroan, the Khond and the Maler. Generally speaking, in the magic and shamanism of

North and middle India the following elements are to be found: shaman schools or at least some systematic training of the candidates; an initiation; a personal tutelary spirit; a call by a spirit or deity.

4. Among the shamanistic paraphernalia the winnowing fan plays the most important role. The winnow is an ancient element in the culture of the Munda peoples. Just as the Siberian shaman brings on his trance by beating his drum, the magicians of North and Middle India try to achieve the same result by shaking rice in the winnow. This explains the total absence of the drum in Central and North Indian shamanism. The winnow has almost the Same function (p. 733).
5. Among many tribes in India, the Shaman calls back the dead person's soul between the third and tenth day after death. But there is no evidence of the typical Altaic and Siberian shaman's ritual of accompanying the souls of the deceased to the land of the dead.

Rahmann concludes saying that, "shamanism essentially consists in a specific relation to a tutelary spirit, which is manifested by the spirit's taking hold of the shaman as its medium, or by its entering into the shaman to invest him with higher knowledge and powers, above all with dominion over other spirits" (p. 751). This definition applies admirably to the characteristics of Middle and North Indian Shamanism, but it does not seem to fit other forms of shamanism (Central and North Asian).

Writing about Shamanism in South India, Harper (1957: 267) refers to shamanism reported by 1931 Census of India with this comment: "On the smallest provocation they (the inhabitants of Malnad in Mysore State) resort to the quack who utters manthras and make sacrifices to the chowdi or to other jungle deity". According to Harper (1957: 268), a shaman in this South Indian: setting is a man who has a familiar-spirit that he can ask to possess him whenever he desires. To achieve a state of possession a certain amount of ritual is gone through, in which the most important element is bathing, after which the familiar-spirit is worshipped, and finally asked to "come on" the shaman. When this happens the shaman goes into a trance and the spirit speaks through him. Many shamans do this at a time, most often once a week. The purpose of the shamanistic possession is to allow people in the human world to have advice and help from a superhuman being whose knowledge and ability to accomplish certain ends is superior to that of any human. "Most shamans control local spirits... who may have a crude stone as a locus of residence. These local spirits often accept or demand blood sacrifice, and not infrequently are accused of causing harm. Each shaman's familiar-spirit has certain idiosyncrasies that belong to him alone and by which he is identified. Most shamans have peculiarities of speech when possessed, perhaps speaking in a 'falsetto singing1 voice or punctuating much of their speech by periodic belching or gasping" (pp. 269-270).

Andaman and Nicobar Islands

According to Radcliffe-Brown (1922:175) in the northern Andaman islands the medicine man is called oko-jumu, meaning dreamer or one who speaks from dreams. The spirits are encountered directly in dreams or in the jungle from whom he obtains all his powers. The medicine men maintained their reputation by the efficiency of their cures and their meteorological magic (for it was they who were believed to foresee storms). But treatment proper consisted in prescribing remedies already familiar to, and used by, every one. Some times, they went on to expel the demons that caused the illness; or again, they promised to finish the cure directly in dreams. The spirits revealed to them the magical properties of various objects including mineral substances and plants. They do not use quartz crystals.

The extremely interesting shamanic initiation is found only in Car Nicobar; it is unknown in the rest of the Nicobar Archipelago. Certain elements are indubitably archaic (the burial under leaves, the withdrawal to the 'land of the spirits'), but many others show Indian influence (the novice's thrown, the lance, the scepter, the staff). We here have a typical example of the hybridization of a shamanic tradition as the result of cultural contacts with an advanced civilization that has elaborated A highly complex magical technique.

The Shaman in the Eastern Ghats of India

The Eastern Ghats (mountain ranges) in South India are a long chain of broken hills and crystalline metamorphic rocks and have a line of mountain ranges running from few meters to 1750 meters height at Biligiri Rangam hills forming their southern tip in Tamilnadu State. These Eastern Ghats are spread over three States viz., Orissa, Andhra Pradesh and Madras and these hilly-forest areas are inhabited by a number of different tribes. Of the 33 scheduled tribes in Andhra Pradesh, 27 live in Eastern Ghats. Some of the predominant tribes of the North Coastal Andhra Pradesh are: the *Bagata, Gadaba, Jatapu, Savara, Porja. Khond, Konda Dora, Valmiki,* etc. They all share the same eco-system and eke out their living either by clearing and cultivating small hilly tracts (shifting cultivation, locally called *'Podu'*) or by working as labourers/coolies in the public works undertaken by the Government. Each of these tribes has their own distinct culture and they are mostly endogamous. There are single tribe villages as well as multi-tribe villages in these Eastern Ghats.

Systematic studies conducted on these tribes demonstrated distinct cultural differences among these tribes. Although cultural differences abound some similarities in the area of Religion is not uncommon. Tribal religion in these parts of India is mostly animistic although the influence of Hinduism is seen in some religious practices. Invoking divine beings for blessings is a common practice at the time of agricultural operations, i.e, sowing and harvesting. In the area of Health too dependence on divinatory forces is distinctly visible in their curative practices. The tribals believe that different elements, conditions, and persons are responsible for different types of ailments. They are natural causes, breach of taboo and social regulations, ancestral spirits, sorcerers and witches, malevolent spirits etc.

The medicine man is locally called as *Yejjodu/Yejjuralu* in Srikakulam district (Rajpramukh, 1976) and Guru or Goragadu etc., in Visakhapatnam district. The medicine man is a part time magico-religious specialist adept at trans-divination, curing by magical power directly from a supernatural source. An important element of the shaman's work is the performance of public (rather private) rituals, in which divination and curing are accomplished through trance. When sickness is not cured for many days the patients approach the Shaman for cure, who is familiar with local medicinal herbs, trees, barks, and pastes made out of crushed leaves. Warding of devils and demons is their specialty and a typical tribal believes in the existence of these spirits and spirit possession of individuals. They also believe in black magic and the first bout of sickness is suspected to be the handiwork of a shaman.

For them spirits are of two kinds: There are malevolent spirits as well as benevolent spirits. Spirits become malevolent, when they were not appeased properly by performing the death ceremony. It could be due to negligence in the performance of the death ceremony or due to defective performance of the ceremony. The malevolent spirits are not propitiated but are feared with repulsion. They try to counter and tame them with the help of the Shaman.

The evil spirits are called by different names (a long list): *Bhoots, Graha peeda, Shanipeeda, Vanukulapeeda, maavelli, Telia Maavelli, Kondapeeda, Geddapeeda, Balagraham, Chandapeeda, Dumbapeeda, Chinugula Dumba, Konda dumba, Adavi peedalu, Sokudu peedalu, Puli bhootham, Chettu bhootham, and Kateru bhootham*. They believe that the evil spirits have the ability to appear in any form—in the form of a man or woman, with the feet pointing backwards and they look like a dazzling glow or a flame emitting sparks.

The favourite abodes of these evil spirits are believed to be trees, stones, old houses and hills. They can travel in air without being seen. Their: most favourite haunting places are burial grounds and natural springs. They can be seen during nights and in twilight. The shaman of Visakhapatnam district believes that there is no hierarchy among these spirits. He asserts that he can confine and release spirits by his magical spells.

The Shaman's Diagnostic Techniques

According to the Shaman, whenever any person is possessed by these evil spirits, the person's pulse becomes very weak and his/her hands become as cold as ice and the patient looks restless. The first step the Shaman initiates is to place a winnow containing burnt cow dung cake over the head of the patient. He then writes the name of a popular god on this cow dung ash. Then invoking the name of his *Guru* (teacher), he chants some mantras to propitiate his spirit-familiar. Thus he commissions his spirit-familiar into the ash which now becomes sacred powder (*vibhoothi*) and smears it on the forehead of the patient. Then he takes a handful of this sacred powder and blows it over the head of his patient. Immediately it is believed that the evil spirit leaves the patient and the patient regains full consciousness. If the spirit still refuses to leave the patient, the shaman mixes pepper powder with the Juice extracted from *Tulasi* leaves and smears it on the eyes of the patient. This medication causes burning sensation in the eyes and tears roll down the eyes of the patients relieving the spirit too. In this haunted condition the patient also would be able to reveal the name of the spirit when his little finger's nail is pressed hard.

If the sickness is due to sorcery or witch craft, the shaman performs a prayer to invoke his spirit-familiar and decides the course of treatment. It is also believed that the spirits of the dead ancestors also appear in the dreams of either the patient or the shaman and are inform them of the mode of treatment to be followed.

The shamans in this region also use talismans. They tie them around their patient's neck or upper hand, even after warding off the evil spirits, to protect them from a relapse of ghost-haunting. The shamans also claim that they also protect houses from being haunted by evil spirits. Chanting of magical incantations is the first step they resort to, followed by fixing nine wooden nails in the nine corners of the house. His magical spell commissions the services of his spirit- familiar to drive away the ghost and the nine nails never allow the ghost to re-enter the house. The shaman, in order to be very effective, has to observe many taboos. He should not light his cigar with other man's lighted cigar. He should not participate in the communal feasts given during the death ceremonies. On Saturdays and Mondays, he is not supposed to eat meat. For his services he never demands any fees. Only voluntary offerings are accepted.

Before taking up the case to cure, the shaman conducts a test or *"Akshintalu Choodadam"* to know whether to take up the case or not. They take a handful of grains (any kind) and count them. If the number is even they know that they can cure the patient and they take up such cases. But if the number is odd, they won't take up the case as they believe that the patient can't survive.

A rather interesting technique is followed to know whether the person is affected by black magic or not. They put some rice in a winnow (or a bowl) and look into the rice with sheer concentration. They maintain that, the image of the black magician, who is responsible for the patient's sickness, appears to him, to him only, in the bowl.

To know whether the patient is affected by ghosts, spirits etc., they make the patient smell a dried herb *'Adavi Pasupu'*. If the patient feels no smell, it is believed that the patient was affected by a ghost. But if he feels a pungent and foul smell, he is considered normal and healthy. They, then use *"Voocha Kommu"* to throw away the evil spirit.

To know what kind of ghost or evil spirit is acting on a patient, they usually feel the pulse *(nadi)*. Some specified parts in the palm have been given names. They hold the wrist of the patient with one hand, and study the points on the palm. At whatever point they feel the change, that point is the ghost, which is said to be responsible for the illness. Then they use the appropriate method to ward off that ghost.

To know the survival chances of a person, bitten by a snake, they crush some kinds of leaves in their palms. If, it produces white foam, they believe that the patient would survive, but if only water comes without foam the patient would, for sure, die. To detect leprosy, they rub the leaves of *Kodimala* on the suspected area of the body. If the patient feels itchy, the skin is normal, but if the patient feels no itching sensation, the skin is supposed to be infected with leprosy.

Treatment for Common Diseases

Many of the common diseases are treated with the locally available herbs, for example, for cold and cough, a powder made of Devadar bark, and locally called *Pherangi chekka* is used. The powder is mixed with water and the patient is made to gulp it. It is believed that this powder helps in better digestion too.

Similarly for whooping cough, the shaman ties a *Raksha* (Talisman) around the neck of the child. This *Raksha* is in the form of a necklace, made out of the fiber of some local tree. If the cough is severe the shaman administers *Tuniki Ginja*. These seeds have to be crushed into a fine powder and some water is added to make it into a fine paste and administered ito the child, orally. For measles, chicken pox etc., the treatment is through the propitiation of local deities. The shaman performs a ritual and uses the flour of *chollu,* turmeric, and some kinds of flowers. During the ritual he chants mantras in front of the fire and throws *Sambrani* (Frankincense) into it. The smoke that emanates is diverted to the body of the patient and is believed to give relief. For epidemics, they sacrifice goats and chicken. In case of dog bites and other wounds, that particular bitten area is bound with a rope made of jute and some crushed herbs with medicinal leaves are placed on it and tied with a cloth. When a person shows unusual symptoms and changes in behaviour and becomes weak gradually in spite of other curative measures, the people believe that he is affected with the *Dumba* (evil spirit). The medicine man possesses innate powers and based on the symptoms identify the particular ancestor of a spirit who is considered responsible for the ill health of the patient. Then he follows a procedure to get in to trance to identify the deceased ancestor and implores it to leave the patient. That procedure requires materials like *'korra'* flour, Sin*dhur,* turmeric powder, *sambrani,* eggs and different types of fruits and flowers. He also chants some incantations. The shaman is paid both in cash and kind. If the patient dies in spite of the shaman's efforts, the blame is passed on only to the powerful evil spirits, but not to the shaman.

The Designs the Shamans Use to Cure Patients

A very interesting feature among the tribes of Eastern Ghats is that the shaman draws different designs for different illnesses, including warding off the spirits or ghosts. Some of the designs they draw for the treatment of different patients are given here under:

For Kateru Ghost

It has 24 corners. This is to be drawn in the burial gtround. With 3 colours red, black, white. At the center the head of A chicken is to be placed and also flowers, green peas etc.

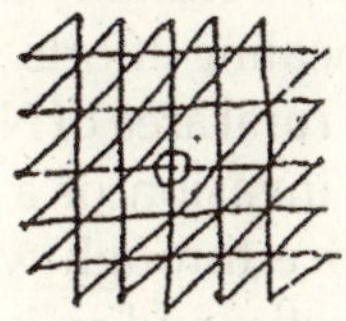

For Shani

This is to be drawn in Thatta. 3 pairs of white flowers, multi coloured chick are required for this. The head of the chick is to be cut down and the blood sprinkled with the head in the design. The Thatta is to be placed at cross roads before 7 AM.

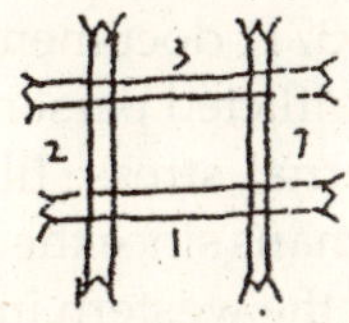

For Dishti Peeda

This is to be drawn in A winnow and is placed in the pathway commonly used.

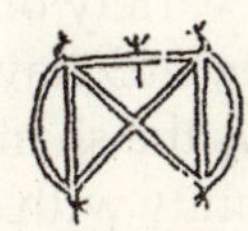

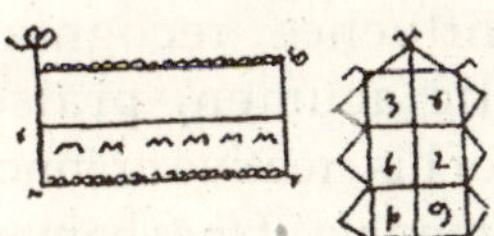

For Dhisti (Evil Eye)

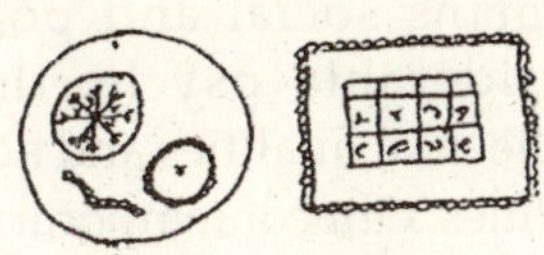

To ward off Ghosts

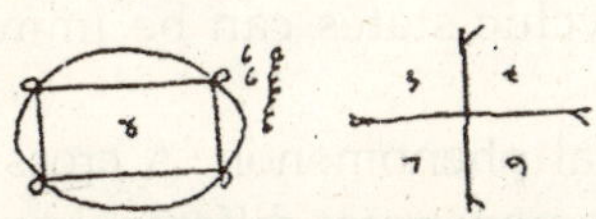

To Drive away Shani (Jinx)

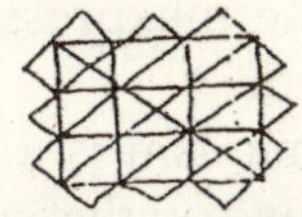

For Rahuvu (Bad times)

Around the four corners of the design or *muggu,* they usually hang pieces' of cloth. In the design or *muggu,* they (the shamans) usually use eggs, the head of a fowl, head of a dove in case of tribes like the *Khond* or *Samantulu,* but for *Bagathas* they use only flowers and chick.

Shamans generally specialize in 'spirit illness' and an important characteristic of many shamans is their ability to go into a voluntary and controlled trance during their diagnostic or healing efforts. Opler (1958) writing on the spirit possession in a rural area of Northern India contends that spirit possession, the invasion of a person by a controlling spirit, is a cultural device through which people can project their psychological anxieties and enlist the support of others. Freed and Freed (1979: 357-371) documented how spirit possession works to reduce the afflicted person's anxiety associated with both internal and external stress. Jilek (1971), summarizing the literature, on shamans since the beginning of this century has demonstrated that the western image of the shaman is full of contradictions. "On the one hand he is seen as 'a mentally ill person' to whom a wide variety of psychiatric labels, like, 'a veritable idiot', 'a trickster,' etc., have been attached". The other side of the picture portrays the shaman as a religious specialist who connects his community with every thing that is sacred and gives meaning to life. He is the mediator between the supernatural and the community. Recent Anthropological literature mentions the shamans social and political influence, recognizes his considerable psycho-therapeutic acumen, praises his intellectual qualities and admiring of his creative or innovative qualities. Our contemporary understanding of the shaman owes much to the influential work of Claude Levi-Straus, who pointed out that the shaman provides the sick member of his society with a language by means of which unexpressed or otherwise inexpressible psychic states can be immediately expressed.

Shamanism is a universal phenomenon. A cross-cultural perspective on this subject demonstrates differences as well as similarities. Available data on Indian tribes exhibits certain striking similarities with shamanism in the Asia-Pacific region.

The most noteworthy is the use of a 'winnow' by the shamans besides trance divination and shamans speaking unintelligible "mantras". A unique feature of the Eastern Ghats tribes is the drawing of various designs by the shamans, deciphering of which would be a rich harvest for those working in the area of Religion and Magic.

Shamanism invariably involves invoking of the supernatural beings as it is universally believed that all illnesses are the result of supernatural wrath and appeasement of these supernatural beings bring back normal state of health. It is also believed in the tribal world that a particular disease is caused by a particular god or goddess. It is firmly believed by the shaman that the cause and cure are located in the same source. The following is an account of such gods and goddesses who are associated with the cause and cure of the diseases.

8

THE HEALING GODS AND GODDESSES

The role of gods and goddesses in curing diseases is universally acknowledged in a variety of cultures since times immemorial. Even in the developed world, especially among the tribal societies such appeasement of gods and goddesses associated with specific illnesses is observed. Such healing gods and goddesses in different cultures are described in the following pages. The local Shaman mediates between the supernatural and the patient.

The Healing Gods and Goddesses

It is interesting to note that in different varieties of cultures people appease and pray numerous gods and goddesses believing that specific bouts of illnesses and epidemics are caused by these supernatural beings. Invoking for the blessings of these gods and goddesses for the cause of the illness is still found in civilized societies also. It is common knowledge in every religion for such a practice even though highly competent physicians attend the patients. Such of these things act as complementary to each other: the physicians treatment and the prayers offered to the supernatural. The following is the list of gods and goddesses in different cultures related to health and disease. A few other gods and goddesses not directly related to health and disease are also given in the list.

Gods and Goddesses of Africa

Aja	Forest Goddess of the Yoruba people. Teaches the use of medicinal herbs.
Gamab	The bushmen call him Gauna and among the Khoikhoi he is known as Gaunab. God of fate and the master of life and death. The supreme deity of the Haukoin people of southern Africa. He shoots arrows from the high heavens at Earth, and those who are hit must die.
Gunab	The Khoikhoi god of evil.
Mbomba	Creator god and ancestral deity of the Mongo people. He is master of life and death. The sun, moon, and man are his children. He is also known as Nzakomba.
Mukuru	The ancestral god and creator god of the Herero bushmen of Namibia. He shows his compassion by providing the rain, caring for the elderly, and healing the sick.
Shakpana	Angry god of the Yoruba, who inflicts man with pox and madness.
Tsui	Khoikhoi god of rain, thunder and sorcerers.

Gods and Goddesses of the Aztecs

Chalchiutotolin	God of pestilence.
Ixtlilton	God of healing, medicine, feasting and games.
Malinalxochi	Sorceress Goddess with power over scorpions, snakes and other stinging, biting insects of the desert
Patecatl	God of healing and fertility

Celtic Gods

Grannus	Healing
Math Mathonwy	Sorcery

Chinese Gods and Goddesses

Yuan-shi tian-zong	"Celestial Venerable of the Primordial Beginning", literally the creator of all things in Heaven and earth. Considered eternal, limitless and invisible.
Yu-huang	The Jade Emperor of Chinese mythology, he rules over all of heaven and Earth. His administrators are the Cheng-huang and Tu-di, as well as other deities in charge of wind, rain, thunder, love, war, etc. The most powerful and revered of Chinese gods.

Gods and Goddesses of the Egyptians

Aker	God of the earth and the dead. Guards the place where the eastern and western horizons meet, as well as the gate through which the pharaoh enters the underworld.
Andjety	God of the underworld, responsible for the rebirth of souls in the afterlife.
Apep	God of chaos, darkness and evil. He battles with the sun god Re">Re to keep the sun from returning to the world

on its nightly journey through the underworld.

Ba — Ram god and a god of fertility. Invoked by women in the hopes that he would help them conceive.

Bat — Cow Goddess of fertility. Pictured as a cow or as a woman with the ears and horns of a cow.

Bes — Grotesque dwarf god. Said to guard households against evil spirits and misfortune. Also a god ofjoviality, dancing, singing and happiness.

Beset — Female version of the god Bes.

Buto — Snake Goddess of the oracle at Buto and protector of the Egyptian royal family.

Ennead — Council of the gods, specifically those of the Osiris pantheon.

Har-nedj-itef — Form of the god Horus. Protector of the dead.

Har-pa-khered — Horus as a child. Invoked to ward off dangerous creatures. Known as Harpocrates by the Greeks.

Hedetet — Scorpion Goddess.

Heket — Goddess of childbirth and protector of the dead. Seen as a frog or a woman with the head of A frog.

Hemsut — Goddess of fate.

Hike — God of supernatural powers. Doctors were called priests of Hike because they invoked the deity during their work.

Horus — Name for a number of gods, all of which invoke thesun, kingship and victory. Horus in his many forms was a protector and warrior god, and the sun and moon were considered his eyes. He was often pictures as a hawk or hawk-headed man.

Imiut — Protective deity of the underworld.

Imset — One of the four protective deities of embalming. Protected the liver of the deceased.

Ipet — Goddess of childbirth and 'mother of the two lands'. Pictured as a hippopotamus.

Isis — One of the most popular goddesses of Egypt. The divine queen and mother of the heavens, both sister and wife to Osiris and mother of Horus. She was the protector and mother-figure of the pharaohs and the protector of women, children and sailors.

Kebechsenef — One of the four gods of embalming. Protector of the lower viscera of the deceased.

Khem — God of fertility, agriculture and human reproduction. Pictured as a mummy.

Mendes — Nature god.

Mesenet — Egyptian Goddess of childbirth. She forms the child in the womb and the ka, or spirit, of the child. Also seen as Goddess of fate or fortune.

Meskhenet — Goddess of midwives and the birth chamber.

Min	God of fertility, vegetation and male virility. Often evoked at the coronation of the pharaoh to ensure his sexual prowess and production of a male heir. Seen as a man holding a flail in his right hand and his erect penis in his left.
Mnewer	Sacred black bull of the sun. Worshipped for his fertility and oracles. Pictured with the solar disk between his horns.
Nekhbet	Vulture Goddess of Upper Egypt and protector of the infant pharaoh. She was present at the birth of the future rulers of Egypt. Pictured on the pharaoh's crown.
Nephthys	'Mistress of the House". Goddess who meets andteaches the newly dead, as weli as comforting the members of their family left alive. Also involved with childbirth. Seen as A woman or a Kite (bird).
Osiris	Important god of Egypt. Seen as the god of thedead and the underworld, although worshipped as a god of fertility, resurrection and vegetation. Married to the sky-Goddess Isis. Killed by his brother Set and chopped into pieces. The pieces were found by Isis and reformed, and he was mummified and resurrected. Re,the father god, did not allow him to stay in the land of the living, but sent him to the Underworld to be thegod and judge of the dead. Seen as a mummified man.
Sakhmet	Also known as Sekhmet. Bloodthirsty and violent Goddess of war and divine vengeance. She is seen as the Goddess who accompanies the pharaoh into battle,as well as the Goddess of plague and disease. Pictured as a woman with the head of A lioness.

Greek Gods and Goddesses

Apollo	One of the Olympian Gods. God of Light, Poetry, Truth, the Arts, Healing and Music. Son of Zeus and Leto. He was an exceptional archer and the God of Oracles. He drives a chariot bearing the sun across the ky each day. Twin brother of the Goddess Artemis. His tree is the laurel, his animal the dolphin, and his bird the crow.
Asclepius	A God of Healing, who perfected the art learned from Chiron. Son of Apollo. His symbol is the snake.
Hygienia	Goddess of Health, closely identified with the worship of Asclepius.

Gods and Goddesses of the Inca

Cocomama	Goddess of health, wealth and happiness.
Supay	God of death and the lord of the Underworld.

Japanese Gods and Goddesses

Binzuru-Sonja	God of curing illness and good vision.
Ekibiogami	God of plagues and epidemics.

Hoso-no-Kami	God of smallpox.
Ukemochi	Goddess of fertility and food.
Yama-no-kami	Goddess of the hunt, forest, agriculture and vegetation.
	Roman Gods and Goddesses
Caia Caecilia	Deified mortal princess Tanaquil.
Meditrina	Sister of Hygeia, daughter of Aesculapius; restored health, whereas Hygeia preserved health; festival in October.
Minerva Medica	Goddess of physicians; Greek Athena.
Valentia	Umbrian town of Oriculum.
Angitia	Healing:especially of poison Sister of Circe and Medea; sacred grove on Lake Fuscinus where both poisonous snakes and medicinal herbs were found.
Clitumnus	Umbrian.
	Gods and Goddesses of the Hindus
Aditya	Twelve sun gods who represent the twelve months of the year. They protect against various diseases and belong to the Devas. They are: Ansa, Aryman, Bhaga, Daksha, Dhatri, Indra, Mitra, Ravi, Savitri, Surya, Varuna, and Yama.
	Gods and Goddesses of Eastern Ghats Tribals
Korangi Gurdi	Chills and fevers; diseases originate from the hills and gales.
Bhima Gurdi	Bites of poisonous lizards and insects.
Gangamma Debta	Measles; general welfare.
Jhanker Debta	Diseases of the forest; ill-health due to eating poisonous leaves, fruits and nuts.
Gorob Nisani	Fevers, weakness affecting resistance due to Jal kamni.
Peda Ammavaru & Chinna Ammavaru	Small pox; Chicken pox.
Kannibhojan	Psychic disorders.
Gusada	Vomitings.

Ethno-Medicine

Administration of local ethno-medicine, supplements the appeasement of the supernatural in curing the illnesses and in warding off the spirits. Tribal cultures, therefore, are the citadels of knowledge related to ethno-medicine. Studies in this area focus on non-western medical systems and the beliefs related to health and illness. A number of Anthropological studies dealt with the general beliefs and definitions of illness. Khare (1963) dealt with medical beliefs held by Gopalpur villagers and stressed the fact that these beliefs quite often link with contrasting medical systems. Some ethno-medical studies have dealt with the functional role of traditional medicines in particular cultures, others have emphasized the logic behind the ethno-medicines; some others have offered the psychological and psycho-somatic implications of these medicines (Bhasin and Srivastava,1991: 9).

Ackernecht (1942a, 1942b, 1943, 1945, 1947 and 1971) was a pioneer in the study of ethno-medicine. Tracing the relationship between primitive medicine and patterns of culture, he identified three important aspects: (i) there is not one but numerous different 'primitive medicines"; (ii) The differences between the primitive medicines are much less in elements than differences in the medical pattern which they build up and which is culturally contained; and (iii) the degree of integration of different elements of medicine to the whole and of the whole medicine into a cultural pattern varies considerably.

Ethno-medicine among the Eastern Ghats Tribals

Field researches in different parts of India have yielded a rich body of data on ethno-medicine. In the Visakhapatnam agency area of Andhra Pradesh different herbal medicines are used for various illnesses. In Araku valley a small plant, *kukkuru mutha (Elephantopus scaber)* root is used to make a decoction and this is administered to patients suffering from joint pains. Among the Porjas, a small herb, *'pedda loyi, (Eupharbia nirifolia)* is used for different purposes. For eye infections the milk of this herb mixed with ash is applied. This treatment also is given to their animals. This application is also administered for back ache. The Shaman in *Gudem Kotha Veedhi* (a tribal village) administers two doses of the ground root of *'seema theega, (sisampalus pareera)'* mixed with water for treating throat pain and constipation. Among the khonds a fern, rama bhanam *(hemonitis arifolia)* leaf is ground with water and is given to those suffering from cough. When taken with milk it rejuvenates the patient with new vigour. In East Godavari District among the tribals, wild onion *(Argenia indica)* is widely used to treat lesions and boils. It is ground into a fine paste and applied to hair to get rid of lice. The bark of *'Billa chettu, (chlorozytis sweetinia)* is used for stomach pain. The root of *kasivinda (kesia occidentalis)* with the root of turmeric *(curcuma longa)* is given in three doses to treat white discharge (leucaria) among the women. For snake bites, the root of *pathala garuda (Rawulfia serpentina)* together with the roots of *sahadevi (verninia synera)* and *nalla easwari (arishtalokhia indica)* is ground into fine powder and a decoction is made with black peppers and orally administered to the patient hourly 10 ml. One most important thing to be observed by those who are present there is while the patient is being treated no one should smoke cigars around that place.

Among the savaras and jathapus of Srikakulam district the *yejjodu* (shaman) uses different roots like *jogigirada (clirodendrum serretum), vepa patta (ajada raktha), naga saram (arishtalokhia indica)* for worm infestations in children. For colds *kukkoti seeds (cleom viscoja)* powder is used.

Among the Konda Reddy, Koyas and Valmikis of West Godavari district, the vadde or vaidyakudu (the medicine man or shaman) uses the bark of oodugumanu (elangium salvifolium) for cough as an expectorant. For body pains the barks of *anem tree (bridelia rituza), bhootha vegisa(kesine glouca), garugudu (garuga pinneta), uciri manu (phyllanthus emblica)* are used.

Among the Konda Doras of Vizianagaram, the Shaman uses the barks of *kothi korandam (mymoja rubikoulis), gotti (jijifus zylopyrus), parimi (jijifus enoplia), billa (chlorozylan sweetinia)* for pains in the waist and legs.

Hemadri's (1994) work on the tribal medicine in coastal Andhra districts is a very interesting and significant contribution and for further references his account gives an elaborate understanding of the tribal medicine in Andhra Pradesh.

9

PARADIGMS OF HEALTH: CONTEXTS OF MARGINALIZATION

Paradigms are developed by social scientists in the area of health and disease. The second half of twentieth century witnessed a paradigm shift with the corporatisation of health care. As a consequence, a large proportion of population is increasingly marginalized in countries like India. The already marginalized underprivileged groups inevitably become further marginalized in this process.

Health is an area of research interest for many disciplines including Anthropology. Social scientists over a period of time developed various paradigms of health. Broadly speaking a paradigm is an example, a conceptual framework within which scientific theories could be generated. A paradigm is a model of truth or a prevalent and accepted way of going about things. Historically, the growth of scientific knowledge has been impeded by paradigms that once worked well but increasingly fail to explain new observations.

In this context, the focus of Health Paradigms is to enable people to confront a situation that is inherently confusing, confounded by the emergence of new innovations and to impart training upon them for leadership roles to handle such situations.

Paradigm Defined

A Paradigm is defined as 'the resilient, inter-locking set of beliefs that literally controls the perception and behaviour of actors in given historical periods. The scientist's paradigm in a particular place and time organically relates every feature of 'reality' in a seamless structural matrix. Those who share a paradigm literally 'see' the world through it, their cognitions, and even their visual intake being fully conditioned by the system of shared beliefs. Reality is relative, systemic, and subjective, not neutral, fragmented or positivistically objective (Marxist Perspectives).

The popular health paradigm is based upon the *medical model*, which is symptom-orientated (physicians treat patients on the basis of symptoms). It is also fragmented and dissociated, with many specialists in the medical system.

The Wellness Model

Medical science, according to many antiestablishment writers, is under attack because it has lusted after the means to health and ignored the ends. In simple terms, writers such as Illich (1974) argue that as the institutions of medicine pursue their own objectives-security, income, growth-they create widespread dependency on the part of the health consumer. Ivan Illich's 'Medical Nemesis' is a powerful critique of the medical establishments. He challenged the fundamental premise of medical 'progress', arguing that institutional medicine is overwhelmingly pathogenic and actively 'sickening'.

The 'Theory of Gaze' formulated by Foucault (1975) is one of the most radical theoretical formulations in which he traces historically how the medical system in the west has operated in the feudal capitalist environment and eventually made the medical profession as an industry–by dehumanizing it. More often than not, the physicians tended to reduce the patient as a specimen of laboratory experimentation.

Although thought to deal with health, medicine actually deals with disease. Over time, it has become more microscopic and reductionistic, able to treat acute diseases successfully, but tending to leave the problem of chronic diseases to the patient and the polity (Carlson, 1975). With the recognition that there are limits to health care growth there is a growing realization of a paradigm shift in medicine. Concepts are changing so that general wellness, rather than the absence of disease, is becoming the standard measure of good health. Medicine is adjusting to such concept changes, albeit quite slowly.

People have tended to think themselves as healthy if they are not in pain, or suffering from cold or flu symptoms, or otherwise impaired in any way that impedes "normal functioning". Under the wellness model, however, health is much more. Abundance of energy, constructive and nurturing relationships, an integral life style, a confident sense of purpose, and the ability to have fun are the optimal dimensions of health.

The wellness model centers on a life style that promotes vitality far beyond what is recognized as feasible in traditional medical circles (MacNeil and Teague, 1987). It should not be confused with holistic health. Holistic health is treatment oriented though it prefers non-surgical, non-drug methods of healing. In contrast the wellness model uses a life style approach that focuses on teachable moments when people are willing to hear and act on the messages their bodies are sending them (Ardell and Tager, 1982). Public sanitation, immunization, hygiene education, physical fitness, nutritional awareness, environmental sensitivity and stress management become part of the wellness model.

It may be noted that paradigms could be of many types depending on the context. The new paradigms of health are more holistic, looking at the person as a whole and the treatments, therefore, are more energy-based and seek to balance the individual, which in turn leads to better health as it addresses the cause of symptoms to allow a longer-lasting improvement in health, rather than simply suppressing symptoms which can arise again later on.

Paradigms of Alternative Medicine

The number of complementary and alternative medicines (CAMs) being utilized by health care consumers is growing at an astounding rate. There is a need by both health care providers and consumers to categorize CAM in order to make meaningful comparisons and informed decisions on their use. Tataryn (2002) proposed four paradigms of health and illness that classify medicines according to the basic assumptions of health and disease associated with each medicine. CAMs classified in the *body paradigm* are those that work through biologic mechanisms, or in other words, target biologic factors as the primary determinants of health (based on ayurveda, homeopathy). The *mind-body paradigm* extends the body paradigm to include factors such as stress, psychologic coping styles, and social supports as primary determinants of health and disease(based on psycho-analysis, psychiatry). The *body-energy paradigm* assumes health and disease are functions of the flow and balances of life energies (based on pranic healing and the Chinese concepts of 'chi' or 'qi'). The *body-spirit* paradigm assumes that one or more transcendental aspects or personalities existing outside the limitations of the material universe can influence health and disease (based on faith healing).

Health Education Paradigms

Jensen (1997) outlines two different paradigms which influence school health education. The first of these is the *moralistic paradigm* which is dominant in many health education programmes in the western schools. It may be argued that the moralistic and totalitarian paradigm may actually be an obstacle for developing a democratic school in a democratic society. The second *paradigm focuses on democratic health education* and is advocated as a valuable alternative to the moralistic paradigm. An overview of the major characteristics of the two paradigms is followed by an analysis of several concepts which characterize democratic health education, including 'action competence', 'action' and 'holism'. These concepts illustrate that health and environment have to be closely linked in teaching if students are to acquire a coherent understanding of the dynamics behind health issues and health problems.

Disease-Specific Paradigms

In the evolution of infant health in Costa Rica two paradigms were identified. One developed in the decades before 1970 and the other during the 1970s. In 1982 Costa Rica had an infant mortality of 18 per 1000 live births and a life expectancy at birth of 76 years for women and 72 years for men. The first or *"malnutrition paradigm"* was orthodox in its derivation; it identified the lack of food as the underlying base for the major health problems and placed its emphasis on institutional medicine. The paradigm was influenced by foreign schools of nutrition and pediatrics and led to the development of an infrastructure for the delivery of medical services and the programs for food distribution. The *"infectious disease paradigm"* recognized infectious diseases as the main determinants of morbidity, mortality and malnutrition in childhood. The strategies derived from such a revolutionary paradigm aimed at the control and eradication of infectious diseases, and they resulted in a rapid improvement of child nutrition and health. However, the infectious disease paradigm does not seem to reduce infant mortality significantly. The necessity of conceptualizing a third new paradigm compatible with health needs of the present and the immediate future is recognized (Mohs, 1985). Thus the *"holistic health paradigm"* is proposed in which the control and prevention of infectious diseases are maintained but priority is given to the prevention of perinatal problems, noninfectious diseases, and various disabilities. This paradigm copes with lifestyles, individual responsibility, and coordination of public and private health and medical care. The paradigm concentrates on emerging health problems that previously were not apparent or were masked by the prevalence of malnutrition and infectious diseases. The dramatic results observed in Costa Rica and in a few other tropical countries demonstrate that health can be improved without undergoing urbanization and industrialization.

New situations develop and along with them new paradigms also are developed. With the corporatisation of health care new paradigms are generated.

Corporatisation of Health Care

This process was initiated and established in the U.S.A., to be replicated later by many other countries including developing countries like India. A new era in American health care can be said to date from 1968 (Light,D.W,1986). In that year Thomas F. Frist and Jack C. Massey–the former a Nashville doctor and the latter the man who had made Kentucky Fried Chicken into a national chain-formed the Hospital Corporation of America (HCA) to provide Frist's private hospital, Park View, with capital for extension. HCA soon began acquiring additional hospitals, and it is now the country's largest investor owned hospital chain.

The juxtaposition of the commercial ethos familiar in fast-food chains with hospital care challenges traditional images of medicine as the embodiment of humane service and even charity. The investor-owned chains have elicited a number of specific criticisms as well, voiced most powerfully by figures in academic medicine such as Arnold S.Relman, professor of medicine at the Harvard Medical School and editor of the New England Journal of Medicine. He and others believe commercial considerations could undermine the responsibility of doctors towards their patients, conceivably leading to unnecessary tests and procedures or-given other financial incentives-to inadequate treatment. Critics of for-profit chains also suspect they drive up the cost of health care, reduce its quality, neglect teaching and research and reject those who can not pay for treatment. This tendency inevitably marginalizes the traditional values of service and charity associated with the health care services. It also tends to marginalize certain professional activities like teaching and research.

By the mid–1960's, physicians, hospitals, private insurers and the government had devised a system of health care financing that was ripe for big business. The form it took–the investor-owned hospital chain-reflects a further condition: the chronic need of hospitals for capital to expand, renovate or equip their facilities. Multi-hospital corporations, unlike privately owned independent hospitals started raising capital by issuing stock.

The Marketplace

To succeed in the market participants must place economic considerations ahead of the care to their patients and their social responsibilities to the community. They must develop patterns of meaning and justifications which allow them to do this. They must somehow make it legitimate.

The introduction of a corporatised market driven health and aged care *system in the USA* has resulted in a health service which has systematically defrauded government, insurers and patients. The interests of patients have been subjugated to the financial demands of the share market. Patients have been used as the vehicle for generating profit without regard to their welfare or their rights. Marketing has replaced care as the key to success, and the value of stock has replaced it as the measure of success. Health care, a humanitarian service to the community is being turned into a marketable product across the world.

Marketplace Ideology

We are faced with a set of concepts variously called market theory, competition policy, economic rationalism, corporatism, micro-economic reform, managerialism etc. They reflect a paradigm developed in the corporate marketplace. It has appropriated the language we use, the structures of society, and the process of globalisation as its own. It is based on self interest and personal greed and is set in stark conflict with traditional social understandings.

It does not recognise or acknowledge this. Instead it labels and discounts social discordance as due to a fear of change. Instead of confronting the fundamental problems and the evidence of dysfunction it talks of educating the community to its point of view. It often markets a caring face and tries to identify with it. It even supports and contributes to public and humanitarian activities. Those who accumulate great wealth bask in their philanthropy.

It is not that self interest is wrong but that it is unbalanced. It is not that philanthropy is wrong but that it is used to create an illusion which those who identify with the patterns of thinking can use to sustain their illusions. It is not even that a marketplace is wrong. It is that the a pattern of ideas which has some application in the marketplace context has been developed and exaggerated into an ideology similar to the other 20th century ideologies (Tataryn, 2002).

Developing Paradigms

When we talk about frames of interpretation, patterns of thought, or paradigms we are talking about the words we use, the understandings we have, and the everyday theories which determine the way we think. The patterns of understanding which people bring to, or which develop in any situation play a major part in determining how they think and how they behave in that situation. To grasp why people behave in dysfunctional ways we should understand the situations within which they find themselves-the context of their lives. The understandings, which they bring with them as well as those, they have developed in response to the particular context provide the clues to their behaviour.

The new breed of health care provider is a businessman with a business training and experience in other businesses. Praise and affirmation comes from the marketplace. He is unlikely to challenge these fundamental beliefs and applies them to health care. Marketplace success is proof of their validity.

Doctors who work within the older medical culture tend to identify with and more readily move towards the marketplace culture because this is advantageous for them personally.

The Contexts and the Meanings

Paradigms (meaning patterns of understanding) developed in a particular context may either conflict with or be congruent with prior understandings. These prior paradigms may be culturally acquired. They may have developed in other contexts. The conflicts between different paradigms become acute when individuals and groups act out their understanding in their actions.

In the business context the measure of success is money and not care. What happens to those who fail to make money because they have acted within a paradigm which considers it unethical to profit at the expense of those who are vulnerable?

They become eventually marginalized under the overpowering forces of corporate culture.

Conflicting Concepts

To understand dysfunctional behaviour we should consider how individuals and groups respond to conflicts between different paradigms (or understandings). We need to relate this to the psychology of individuals and groups to see how and why some individuals and groups succumb to the pressures surrounding them while others resist-why some individuals succeed in a particular context and others fail.

To understand health care today we need to recognise the conflicts between the marketplace paradigm and the more community orientated and traditional Hippocratic and Samaritan paradigms with which the health care professions and the community have identified. The marketplace paradigm is exemplified in the thrust to "reform" health care using competitive market forces. Proponents of market forces do not acknowledge the conflicts. They have discounted them on the one hand by labeling the health care paradigms as obsolete and criticising those who promote them. On the other they claim a commitment to *care* and *quality* on the basis that the two are congruent and that good care increases profits. Customers, they claim, will ensure this. Market proponents claim that marketplace success is proof of good care. People would not pay for it if it wasn't.

They are not being dishonest. They really believe this. Because the paradigms they use have lost contact with reality they can bend them to whatever purpose they wish without noticing any contradiction.

Post Modernism

There is a new "post modern" intellectual movement. This eschews all embracing theory and sees meaning as integral to context and the way people live. Without denying broad understandings of human behaviour it sees the meanings by which we live as individual and context related. Broad theories may or may not have relevance in a particular context. In other words understandings are seen to relate to particular situations rather than all situations. This movement is young and in a world dominated by an all-embracing corporatised understanding of globalisation it evidently has no power.

The Indian Context: In the area of health planning, the unquestioned shift to privatization, hi-tech medical care, introduction of fees in public hospitals, cuts introduced in public health, specially communicable disease control and water supply, and undermining primary health care (PHC), with undue emphasis on a women-centered Family Planning Programme reflects the lack of intellectual concern about the less-privileged in society. The reasons underlying the shifts are neither logical nor inevitable. They are more often the result of the prevailing colonization of the mind through knowledge born out of a context in which public health as a discipline has become extremely narrow, quantitative, hi-tech oriented and devoid of social and political context (Quadeer, 1995).

The first comprehensive document on health planning produced by the Indian government in 1946 recognized that unemployment and poverty have a profoundly adverse effect on health through the operation of such factors as inadequate nutrition, unsatisfactory housing and clothing, and lack of proper medical care during periods of illness. 'In Independent India, however, health planning assumed that poverty will be tackled by other sectors. It confined itself to building infrastructure and technology-based intervention programmes. It evolved a concept of 'Basic Health services' which included essential inputs such as control of communicable diseases, maternity and child health, family planning, basic curative services, nutrition and health education. By the mid-seventies the failures were evident' (Qadeer, 1995). Later in 1979 the concept 'Primary Health Care' was hoisted by the new government at the centre. This concept was different from Basic Health Care as it attempted to operationalise the later within a socio-economic, political and cultural context. Basic Health service was simply the statement of the minimum medical and public health needs of the people. It recognized the links between lack of nutrition, clean environment, water supply, unemployment and poor infrastructure, and disease but did not necessarily incorporate them in its own operationalisation. Primary Health Care not only achieved this conceptual sophistication but also emphasized the primacy of political and social organizations, perceptions of need and values of the people.

India also was a signatory to the 'Alma Ata' declaration of 'Health for all by 2000' without realizing the mammoth task ahead. Poverty is central to all the problems related to the health of a people in all the un/under-developed countries including India. At the time of Alma Ata declaration in 1978, more than 35% of Indian population was living below poverty line. In a survey (Rajpramukh, 2001) conducted on the tribals of Vizianagaram district in 2001, it was found that infant mortality rate was between 12-15 per 1000 where as the current national figure was 4 per 1000. In some of the primitive tribes like the savaras and porjas it was found to be more than 25 per 1000. So long as poverty is going to be there diseases abound and eradication of poverty in a populous country like India is not an easy task.

Another set back in our policy formulation is that there is absolutely no involvement of the people as our approach invariably is 'top-down'. Besides our policy is always physician/hospital centered but not people/patient centered.

Marginalization of the Marginalized: With the advent of corporatised hi-tech medicine in India and the high costs associated with it the health care delivery in urban areas have witnessed tremendous changes. In urban areas even the large majority of middle class feel marginalized for not being able to utilize the medical services in the corporate hospitals because of the unaffordable high costs. Corporate medicine, thus, becomes the prerogative of the upper class rich only. Another major contributory factor for this malady is that health insurance is not a popular concept with many of the people in India unlike the western countries, where almost every one is covered by insurance. Such a situation leaves a very large majority of the population helpless although highly efficient medical expertise is available within the same society in which they leave.

With regard to the rural and tribal people, the situation becomes much more harsh as they seek low/no cost health care delivery. The poor condition of the Primary Health Centres contribute to their woos and in many places a large proportion of under-utilization of PHCs was reported. In tribal areas the presence of quacks and some native medicine men exacerbate their health problems by resorting to aggressive medication. There are many things to it and the whole process marginalizes the already marginalized further.

Conclusion

Until probably the middle of the 20th century the paradigms which governed the provision of health care required that it be provided only in the interests of the individuals who were ill. Those who provided these services on behalf of society were entitled to a reasonable reward for their services. They were ethically bound to place the interests of the ill person ahead of any personal gain.

During the second half of the 20th century commercial forces increasingly impacted on health care and the professions bent before the winds of change. The consequent dysfunction was seen as due to professionalism itself, rather than the impact of market forces on professionalism. The response was to increase market forces. By the end of the 20th century corporatisation was progressing rapidly and health care was increasingly a servant of the stock market.

The corporatisation of health care is a consequence of a new set of universal economic belief systems which have come to dominate social processes. This new belief system has made it socially acceptable and perfectly legitimate for some members of society to profit economically from the miseries and vulnerability of others. Those who provide care are expected to do so for the economic benefit of corporate groups and of third parties who have no direct interest in the patient's welfare. Care for the patient has been replaced by care for the corporation. Patterns of thinking have been developed to make this socially acceptable. Market theory conflicts directly with norms that have protected vulnerable people from exploitation for over 2000 years.

India still exhibits traditional features as more than 70% of the population still lives in the rural and tribal areas. Indian scenario started exhibiting the same tendencies, mostly in urban centers, associated with the process of corporatisation but with a difference: the difference lies in the vast proportions of populations being marginalized in tribal, rural and even urban contexts.

10

ANTHROPOLOGIST'S ROLE

The basic Anthropological Orientation should offer useful ideas related to health and disease. As Anthropology studies human behaviour which is shaped and conditioned by one's culture, the behaviour and culturological factors are taken into consideration in dealing with matters related to health and disease. As a change agent health education plays an important role in the community life and as Anthropologists have fairly good idea about the natives cultures, they are better equipped than others in imparting health education to bring about desired changes.

Health education is a study in human behaviours in those situations that affect the health of the people. As a profession, it utilizes educational processes to effect change in the health practices of individuals and groups (including families, organizations and communities). Its intent is the generation of behaviour through the explanation of both the options for change as their consequences. It is not a single discipline but a "field of interest" drawing on the contributions of biomedical, biostatistical and behavioural science" (Smith Bryan 1979: 300). As Anthropology combines all the fields in its scope, without doubt it is the well-equipped of all the disciplines in this context.

The aim of health education is to assist people to value health as a quality of life. Its purpose is to help them attain personal goals by utilizing their maximum potential to a better self and community. The objectives are to interest people in their health and the needs to improve it, which, what, and where health care services are available; when to use them; and how to discriminate in making choices for prevention and care (Smith, Bryan 1979: 300).

Health behaviour change is the important goal of health education. Any community health education program meant for controlling a specific disease in a population must be coordinated in the following series of steps:

1. Nature of the problem must be documented including the population at risk.
2. Identify the behaviour change(s) that will result in the reduction of mortality and morbidity.
3. The resources necessary to solve the problem must be identified.
4. Other inter reactions which facilitate change must be utilized.
5. Measurement of the behaviour change as a result of health education program.

As Anthropologists are familiar with the attributes and values of the natives, any behaviour change that is intended to bring about better health status for the community would not have impediments as the natives trust Anthropologists who spent portrayed periods of time among them in their research endeavours. Influencing groups of people is complex process and Anthropologists are adept at this task.

The following key areas would offer significant factors, which highlight relevance of medical anthropology to certain global health problems:

1. Over population
2. Environment (Pollution and Global Warming)
3. Nutrition and hunger
4. Housing
5. Medical care including primary health care

6. Urbanization
7. AIDS
8. Welfare

Primary Health Care

The WHO issued its famous declaration in 1978 at Alma-Ata of 'Health for all by 2000'. This ambitious programme intended to develop, throughout the world, a comprehensive system of Primary Health Care (PHC).

The concept of PHC has provided the framework for health care strategies globally since its formulation at Alma-Ata where it was defined as: "essential health care based on practical, scientifically sound and socially acceptable methods and technology, made available to individuals and families in the community through their full participation and at a cost the community and country can afford to maintain at every stage of their development in the spirit of self-reliance and self-determination" (Abbatt and McMahon 1985:6).

WHO has defined eight components of PHC–health education, nutrition, immunization, maternal and child health, family planning, water and sanitation, control of endemic diseases and treatment of common diseases and provision of essential drugs. Programmes to address these eight components of PHC have developed throughout the world since 1978, varying in emphasis according to temporal and spatial trends. Health education is at the centre of the circle of PHC emphasizing its conceptual importance.

Health Education Models

The following three basic health education models are identified:

1. Knowledge, attitude, behaviour model (KAB)
2. Self-empowerment model
3. Community action model

The original KAB model is based on the now largely discredited theory that new knowledge leads to attitudinal and behavioural change. The model is based on a view of human beings as rational decision-makers and a positivist view of society operating accordingly to universal mechanistic laws. This model is now considered as overly simplistic as knowledge is perceived as only one a member of factors which affect health behaviour.

The 'self empowerment' model of health education is based on the concept of improving health through developing people's ability to understand and control their health status to whatever extent possible within their environmental circumstances.

The community action model is based on the concept of improving health by changing environmental, social and economic factors through community involvement and action. It has developed primarily in response to the failure of earlier health education models.

The role of Anthropologists in Imparting Health Education is crucial. Anthropological methodology makes the researcher as a part of the community as he stays with them for a prolonged period of time. His familiarity will every one in the community helps him to push any development programme into their midst without any resistance. In other words, he can convince the members of the community much better than any one else in promoting any development programme including the health promotion programmes. In all the components of PHC, in order that the programmes end up successfully with 100% acceptance from the people, Anthropologists handle the situation much better than others.

Helman (2001:263) lists the following roles of medical Anthropology in a global health policy:

1. To carry out detailed research in local communities and social groups into the social and cultural dimensions of specific health problems and diseases.
2. To provide a comprehensive database on the social and cultural compassion of different communities world-wide based on prior research by other anthropologists.
3. To study the relationship between health or communities; i.e. to explore the differences between what people

say they believe or do and what they actually do in practice, and explain the reasons for these discrepancies.

4. To mediate between health interventions at the local level and policy makers at the national or international levels in order to adopt the programme to specific local conditions.

5. To aid in these interventions at the local level by:
   (a) ensuring that the programme 'makes sense' to the community, in terms of their local social, cultural and economic realities.
   (b) identifying community resources useful for health education or health care, as part for national or international programme.
   (c) monitoring the impact of these programmes on the local community.
   (d) developing a network of locally recruited "barefoot anthropologists" (research assistants) or social scientists, to assist in the planning, application and evaluation of the programme.
   (e) providing feedback for policy makers on the progress and impact of the programme.
   (f) adapting health education programmes to disseminate information through culturally appropriate channels within the community (such as teachers, religious leaders or traditional healers).
   (g) acting as advocates or culture interpreters, for the community to health bureaucracies and policy makers at the national or international levels.
   (h) To organize educational programmes on the social and cultural dimensions of health and disease for policy makers, and for other researchers.
   (i) To monitor the institutional cultures of national and international medical aid agencies, to improve their efficiency and help reduce ethnocentric bias.

(j) To develop and test new research instruments (such as rapid assessment procedures) to study particular health problems in specific local and national contexts.

New Applied Anthropology

Indigenous knowledge research sets out explicitly to make connections between local peoples understanding and practices and those of out side researchers and development workers, notably in the natural resources and health sectors, seeking to achieve a sympathetic and in-depth appreciation of their experience and objectives and to link them to scientific technology (Sillitoe, 1998). In this context, participatory research techniques have been generated in different social sciences and the main thrust in such an approach is to make the people or the subjects into active collaborators in bringing about desired change. Technology transfer is now considered not as a top – down imposition but as a search for jointly negotiated advances, which results in cost-effective, time-effective programmes generating appropriate insights readily intelligible even to non-experts. Thus participatory approaches seek a more systematic accommodation of indigenous knowledge in research and technological interventions (Schaffer, 1989). The demands of indigenous knowledge and participatory research require the establishment of partnerships founded on dialogue. Anthropologists are better positioned to take up the tasks of incorporating indigenous knowledge into the development process as they are the pioneers in documenting indigenous knowledge systems through participant observation method that involves living with the subjects for a very long period. This being the hallmark of Anthropological research, the role-play of 'Anthropologists as consultants' in implementing development programmes becomes much more relevant compared to other social scientists.

Haile (1996) proposes that the idea of harnessing Anthropology to technical knowledge to facilitate development puts the discipline where it should be, at the center of the development process. This focus on indigenous knowledge has already resulted in reappraising theoretical as well as methodological aspects of Anthropology. The liability of indigenous knowledge is reflected in the theoretical shift from a structural to a processual and to a post-modernist perspective. Certain methodological advances to tailor interventions to local conditions have already been put forward by the Anthropologists in 'doing Anthropology' by a very different process.

The process involves the brokering of knowledge in which Anthropologists become researchers for and consultants to indigenous people and traditional communities (community-controlled research). They can also oversee that the indigenous knowledge is not patented for but used in the production of universal medical technologies, not for private commercial benefits. This will establish the 'dialogue' as the cornerstone of a new Applied Anthropology. In this endeavour, the greatest challenge to Anthropology vis-à-vis development debate is to develop criteria and indicators for sustainable development–health environments, sustainable livelihoods that are based on local, indigenous perceptions, classifications, values, measures of environmental quality and change that reflects local observations and knowledge systems, even if they seem 'magical', whimsical or destructive to the outsider.

REFERENCES

Alland, Alexander Jr. (1966), Medical Anthropology and Bio-cultural Adaptation–Am. Anthrop., 68:40-57.

Alland (Jr.) A. (1970), "Adaptation in Cultural Evolution: An Approach to Medical Anthropology", Columbia Univa. Press, New York.

Abbatt and Mc Mahon (1985), "Teaching Health Care Workers: A Practical Guide", Mac Millan, London.

Ackernecht Erwin H. (1942 a), Problems of Primitive Medicine. Bull. Hist. Med., xi, 503-521.

Ackernecht Erwin H. (1942 b), Primitive Medicine and Culture Pattern. Bull. Hist. Med., xii 545-574.

Ackernecht, E.H. (1945), "On Collecting of Data Concerning Primitive Medicine", *American Anthropology*, 47 : 427-432.

Ackernecht, Erwin H. (1943), "Psychopathology, Primitive Medicine and Primitive Culture", Bull. Hist. Med., xiv : 30-67.

Ackernecht, Erwin H. (1947), Primitive Surgery. Am. Anthrop., 49: 25-45.

Ackernecht, Erwin H. (1971), Medicine and Ethnology: Selected Essays. The Johns Hopkins Press, Baltimore.

Alland, Alexander Jr. (1970), "Adaptation in Cultural Evolution; An Approach to Medical Anthropology", Columbia University Press, New York.

Allison, A.C. (1954), "Protection Afforded by Sickle-cell Trait against Sub-tertian Malarial Infection", Br. Med. J., 1:290

APHA (1985), Standard Methods for the Examination of Water and Waste Water. 16th Edition. New York: American Public Health Association.

Ardell, D.B. and Tager, M.J. (1982), Planning for Wellness. Kendall/ Hunt Publishing Co. Dubuque, IA.

Atran, Scott (1999), Managing the Maya Commons: The Value of Local Knowledge. In Ethno Ecology: Situated knwledge/located lives (ed.) Nazarea University, Amizona Press, Tuejon, pp. 190-214.

Atte, O. (1992), Indigenous Local Knowledge as a Key to Local Level Development: Possibilities, Constraints, and Planning Issues. Ames: Iowa State University.

Barrow, E.G.C. (1992), "Building on Local Knowledge: The Challenge of Agro-forestry for Pastoral Areas", Agro-forestry Today 3(4): 4-7.

Barth, Fredrik (1990), The Guru and the Conjurer: Transactions in Knowledge and the Shaping of the Culture in Southeast Asia and Melanesia. Man, n.s, 25: 640-53.

Barth, Fredrik (2002), "An Anthropology of Knowledge", Current Anthropology, 43(1) 1-18.

Berlin, Brent (1994), "Anthropological issues in Medical Anthropology", Ethnology and the Search for News Drugs (ed). Prance, Ciba Foundation Symposium Publication, 185 .

Berlin, Brent, and Elois Ann Berlin (1994), "Anthropological issues in Medical Anthropology," in Ethnobotany and the Search for New Drugs. Ed. by G. Prance. Ciba Foundation Symposium Publication 185.

Bhasin and Srivastava (1991), "Medical Anthropology: A Review", *Journal of Human Ecology,* 2(I) 1-19 Delhi.

Bhupesh M. (1992), "India Disquiet About AIDS Control", *The Lancet,* Vol. 240, No. 8834/8835.

Blum R. and E. Blum (1965), "Health and Healing in Rural Greece", Stanford University Press, Stanfard.

Blumenhagen (198)), "Hypertension: A Folk Illness with a Medical Name", Culture, Medicine and Psychiatry, 4:197-227.

Blumenhagen (1981), On the Nature of Explanatory Models. Culture, Medicine and Psychiatry, 5:331-40.

Brothwell, D. "Major Congenital Anomolies of the Skeleton" in Diseases in Antiquity: A Survey of Disease Injuries, and Surgery in Early Population (ed.) Sanderson & Brothwell, Springfield.

Brouwer, Jan (1998), On Indigenous Knowledge and Development, in Discussion and Criticism, Current Anthropology, 40(3).

Bunce (1972), Aggravation of Vitamin A Deficiency Following Distribution of Non-filtered Skim Milk: An Example of Nutrient Interaction. The Careless Technology (ed.) Farrer and Milton, Garden City, Natural History Press, pp. 53-60.

Carlson, R.J. (1975), "The End of Medicine", John Wiley & Sons, New York.

Codrington, R.H. (1891), "The Melanesians: Studies in their Anthropology and Folklore, Oxford.

Caudill (1953), Applied Anthropology in Medicine, in Anthropology Today. A.L. Kroeber (Ed.) University of Chicago Press, Chicago.

Chen, E. and N.A. Cobb (1960), Family Structure in Relation to Health and Disease: A Review of the Literature, *Journal of Chron Diseases,* 12: 544-567.

Christensen *et.al.* (1953), "Measles in Virgin Soil", Acta. Med. Scand. 144:430.

Clements, F.E. (1932), "Primitive Concepts of Disease", Barkeley (CPAEE xxx 11, 2).

Colson, and Selby (1974), Medical Anthropology, Ann. Rev. Anthrop., 3: 245-262.

Cotran, S.R. Kumar, V. and S.L. Robbins (1989), Pathologic Basis of Disease. W.B. Saunders Company, Philadelphia, 4th International Edition, Ch. 1, p. 1.

Dasen (1993), "Dwarfs in Ancient Egypt and Greece", Clarendan Press, Oxford.

Deshkar, S., Biswas, S.K. Appulingam, S., Chavan, S., Kashyap, R. Bandopadhyay, S.S. and A.N. Deshmukh (1988), Biochemical Impact of High Fluoride Environment in Fluoride is Affected Subjects of Dhaptala Village, Tahsilkorpana, District Chandrapur Environmental Biochemistry, 1: 25 28.

Dunn, F.L. (1976), Human Behavioural Factors in the Epidemiology and Control of Wuchereria and Brugia Infections. Bull. Public Health, Soc., Malay, 10:34-44.

Dunn, F.L. (1979), Behavioural Aspects of the Control of Parasitic Diseases. Bull WHO, 57:499-512.

Dunn, F.L. (1983), Human Behaviour Factors in Mosquito Vector Control SE Asean. J. Trop. Med. Public Health, 14: 86-94.

Evons, Ivor H.N. (1923), Studies in Religion, Folklore and Custom in British North–Borneo and the Malay Peninsula, Cambridge.

————(1930), Schebesta on the Sacerdo-therapy of the Semang, *J. of Royal Anth. Inst.* London.

Eliade, Mircea (1974), Shamanism: Archaic Techniques of Ecstasy, Bollingen Series LXXVI Princeton University Press.

Elizabeth, K.M., and K.E. Rajpramikh (2000), Potability of Water among the Tribals of Viziangaram Sub-plan Area, Andhra Pradesh: Microbiological and Physico-chemical Analysis: The Anthropologist, 12, 3.

Ellen, R.F. and Harris (1997), "Indigenous Environmental Knowledge in Scientific and Developmental Literature: A Critical Assessment", Canterbury: University of Kent at Canterbury.

Elwin, Verrier (1947), The Muria and their Gotul, Bombay.

————(1949), Myths of Middle India.

————(1955), The Religion of an Indian Tribe, London.

Vans–Pritchard (1937), Witcharaft, Oracles and Magic among Azande. Clarendon Press, Oxford.

Fairhead, J. Rajasekaran and Warren (1991), Indigenous Technical Knowledge and Natural Resources Management in Sub-saharan Africa: A Critical Overview. Kent, U.K.: Natural Resources Institute, Chatham Maritime.

Fischer, Edward F. (1999), Cultural Logic and Maya Identity: Rethinking Constructivism and Essentialism. Current Anthropology, 40: 473-99.

Foster and Anderson (1978), "Medical Anthropology", John Wiley and Sons, New York, Brisbane and Toronto.

Fabrega, Jr. (1972), Medical Anthropology, p. 167–229, in: Biennial Review of Anthropology, B.J. Slegel (Ed). Stand Ford University Press.

Fortune, R.F. (1932), Sorcerers of Dabu, London.

Foucault (1975), The Birth of the Clinic: An Archaeology of Medical Perception Vintage Books, New York.

Foucalt, M. (1972), The Archaeology of Knowledge, London Tavistok

Frank, J.D. (1963), Persuasian and Healing, New York, Schacken Books.

Freed and Freed (1964), "Spirit Possession as Illness in a North Indian Village", Ethnology 3:152–71.

Freed, A and Ruth S. Freed (1979), "Sprit Possession as Illness in a North Indian Village", Issues in Cultural Anthropology (ed.) David W. McCurdy and James P. Spradley, Waveland Press Inc., p. 357-371.

Gagnon (1950), "Contribution to Study of Etiology and Prediction of Cancer of Cernix of Uterns, Am. J. Obstet, Gynecol 60:516.

Good, B.J. (1977), "The Heart of What's the matter: The Semantics of Illness in Iran", Culturals Medical and Psychiatry, 1: 25–58.

Ghosh T.K. (1986), "AIDS: A Serious Challenge to Public Health', *Journal of the Indian Medical Association,* January; 84(1): 29-30.

Haile, J. (1996), "Umbilical, Anthropology in Action", *Journal for Applied Anthropology in Theory and Practice,* 3:52-55.

Helman, C.G. (2001), "Culture, Health and Illness", Oxford University Press, Reprint by Arnold.

Hall, Edward T. (1984), "The Dance of Life", p. 230–31, Anchor Press.

Hallowell (1940), "Aggression in Soubteaux Society, Psychiatry 3: 345–407.

Hamadri, K. (1994), Sastravethalanu Akarshistunna Girijan Vaidyam (Telugu) TCR & TI, Hyderabad.

Handy, E.S.C. (1923), "The Native Culture in the Marquesas", Berenicwe P. Bishop Museum Bulletin 9 (Hanalulu).

Harper, Edward B. (1957), "Shamanism in South India", S.W. *Journal of Anthropology,* XIII pp. 267–87.

Harwood (1970), WITHCRAFT, Sorcery and Social Categories among the Safwas London: Oxford University Press.

Henry and Henry (1944), Zunia: Dal Play of Village Indian Children. American Orthos Psychiatric Association Research Monograph, No. 4

Hesser, J.E. (1982), "Studies of Infectious Diseases in An Anthropological Context", Medial Anthropology, 6: 1-10.

Hoskin *et. al.* (1969), Epilepsy and Guria: The Shaking Syndromes of New Guinea Soc. Sec. Med 3:39–48.

ICMR, (1975), Manual of Standards of Quality for Drinking Water Supplies. Indian Council of Medical Research, Special Report No. 44:27.

Illich, Ivan (1974), "Medical Nemesis", The Lancet, p. 918-921.

Jensen, B.B. (1997), "A Case of Two Paradigms within School Education", *Health Education Research,* Vol. 12, No. 4, 419-428.

Jilek, G. (1971), From Crazy witch Doctor to Auxiliary Psychotherapist, The Changing Image of the Medicine Man, Psychiatry Clinic, 4, p. 200-220.

Keesing, R.M. (1981), "Cultural Anthropology: A Contemporary Perspective", Halt, Rinehart & Winston.

Kakar, Sudhir (1982), Shamans, Mystics and Doctors, Oxford University Press.

Kakar D.N. and Kakar S.N. (2001), "Combating AIDS in the 21st Century Issues and Challenges", Sterling Publishers Private Limited, p. 31.

Kapferer, Bruce (1996), "The Feast of the Sorcerer: Practices of Consciousness and Power", University of Chicago Press-Chicago.

Khare R.S. (1963), "Folk Medicine in North Indian Village", Human Organization, 22.

Kiev, A. (1968), Curanderismo, New York, Frce Press of Glencoe.

Kinsey *et.al.* (1953), "Sexual Behaviour in the Human Female", W.B. Saunders & Co. Philadelphia.

Kleinman, A. (1980), "Patients and Healers in the Context of Culture. An Exploration of the Border Land between Anthropology, Medicine and Psychiatry", University of California Press, Brekeley.

Koch, K. (1968), On 'Possession' Behaviour in New Guinea, *Journal of Polynesian Society,* 77: 135-46.

Kroeber and Kluckhohn (1963), "Culture: A Critical Review of Concepts and Definitions", New York, Vintage Books.

Kulkarni, V.S. (2005), Nutritional Assessment and Evaluation, in Reproductive and Child Health Problems, (ed.) K.K.N. Sarma, Academic Excellence, New Delhi, p. 131-141.

Kunstadter , P. (1962), Discussion of S. Polgars Paper in Health and Disease: A Receive of the Literature, *J. Chron., Diseases,* 12: 544-567.

Latour, Bruno (1987), "Science in Action", Cambridge: Harvard University Press.

Leach, E. (1982), Social Anthropology, p. 38–39, Fontana.

Landy, D. (ed.) (1980), "Culture, Disease and Health: Studies in Medical Anthropology", Mac Millian Publishing Co., Inc., New York.

Langness L.L. (1965), Hysterical Psychosis in the New Guinea Highlands: A Bena Bena Example. Psychiatry, 28 :258-77.

Lewis, I.M. (1966), Spirit Passession and Deprivation Cults, Main 1: 307–29.

Light, Donald W. (1986), Corporate Medicine for Profit, *Scientific Medicine*, Dec., Vol. 255, No. 6, p. 38-47.

Loeb, E.M. (1935), Sumatra: Its History and People.

Mac Mahon *et.al.* (1960), Epidemiologic Method, Little, Brown & Co., Boston.

MacNeil, R.D. and Teague, M.L. (1987), Aging and Leisure: Vitality in Later Life, Prentice-Hall, New Jersey.

Maiti, T.I. (1982), "The Dangerous Acid Rain", *Science Reporter,* 19: 360-36.

Margetts, E.L. (1965), Traditional Yorupa healers in Nigeria, Man, 65 (102).

Mausner and Bahn (1974), Epidemiology: An Introductory Text, W.B. Saunders & Company, Phildelphia.

Miles, Dauglas (1966), Shamanism and the Conversion of Ngadgu Dayaks, Oceamia, Vol. xxxvii, Sept. No.1, p. 1-12.

Millet *et. al.* (1980), Rome: Mummfication for the Common People, Mummies Disease and Ancient Cultures (ed.) Aiden and Eve Cockburn, Cambridge Univ. Press, Cambridge.

Mishler, E. and N.A. Scotch (1964), Socio-cultural Factor in the Epidemiology of Schozophrenia, Psychlatry.

Mohs, E. (1985), Evolution of Paradigms of Child Health in Developing Countries, Pediatric, Infect, Dis. Sept-Oct., 4(5), 532-537.

NACO (2006), HIV/AIDS Epidemiological Surveillance & Estimation Report for the Year, 2005.

Newman, P.L. (1964), 'Wildman' Behaviour in a New Guinea Highland Community, American Anthropologist, 66:1–19.

National Research Council (1972), *Accumulation of Nitrate,* National Academy of Science Washington, D.C., p. 106 (1972).

Nazarea, V. (1999), A View From a Point: Ethno-ecology as situated Knowledge, University of Arizona Press, Tucson.

Nigh, Ronald (2002), Maya Medicine in the Biological Gaze, *Current Anthropology*, 451-77.

Nuckub, C. (1991), "Culture and causes Thinking: Diagnosis and Pracsctian in a South Indian Folky Village, Ethnos 19 (I) 3-11.

Opler, M.E. (1963), The Cultural Definition of Illness in Village India, Hum. Organiz, 22, 32-35.

Opler, M.E. (1958), Spirit Possession in a Rural Area of Northern India, Reader in Comparative Religion (ed.) W.A. Lessa and E.Z. Vogt Evanston, pp. 553-566.

Osborne, O.H. (1969), The Yoruba Village as a Therapeutic Community J. Health. Sec. Behaviour, 10: 187-200.

Preston–Whyte, (1995), Halt-way There: Anthropology and Intervention Oriented AIDS Research in Kwazalu /Natal, South Africa in Culture and Sexual Risk: Anthropological Perspectives on AIDS (ed.) H. Ten Brummalkvis and G. Herdt, pp. 315-37, Gordan and Breach.

Panda S. (2002), "The HIV/AIDS epidemic in India: An Overview", in Panda S., Chatterjee A. and Abdul-Quader A.S. (Eds.), "The Epidemic and the Response in India", p. 20.

Polgar (1962), Health and Human Behaviour: Areas of Interest Common to the Social and Medical Science, *Current Anthropology*, 3: 154-205.

Parsons (1951), The Social System, The Free Press, Glaseve, Illinois.

Paul, B.D. (1963), Anthropological Perspective on medicine and public health. Ann Amer . Acad . P.A. Soc. Sci., 346 :334.

Paul and Rao (2002), Dimensions and Implications of Drug Trafficking and Drug Abuse in India, Social Defense, National Institute of Social Defense Govt. of India, pp. 4-36.

Paul, B.D. (1950), Health, Culture and Community, Russel–Sage Foundation, New York.

Pelczar Jr. Michael J., Chan E.C.S. and N.R. Krieg (1986), Microbiology: New Delhi, Tata Mc Graw-Hill Publishing Company Limited.

Polgar, S. (1962), "Health and Human Behaviour: Areas of Interest Common to the Social and Medical Sciences", *Current Anthropology*, 3 No. 2: 159-205.

Polgar, S. (1964), Evolution and the Ills of Mankind In: Horizons of Anthropology, (ed.) S. Tax, p. 200-2111, Aldine, Chicago .

Press, I. (1969), Urban Illness: Physicians, Curers and Dual Use in Bagota, *Journal of Health Soc. Behaviour*, 10 : 209-18.

Qadeer, Imrana (1995), Primary Health care–A Paradise Lost, *IASSI Qrtly*, Vol. 14, Nos. 1&2, p. 1-20.

Rivers (1924), "Medicine, Magic and Religion", Kegan Paul, Trench, Trubner and Co., London.

Radciffe–Brown, A.R. (1922), "The Andaman Islanders: A Study in Social Anthropology", Cambridge.

Rahmann, Rudolf (1959), "Shanmistic and related Phenomena in Northern and Middle India Anthropos, LIV, pp. 681-760.

Raj Pramukh, K.E. (1976), A Note on the Shaman among the Jatapus, Folklore, 17(2): 379-381.

Rajpramukh, K.E. (2001), Morbidities and Mortalities among the Tribals of Vizianagaram District, Report submitted to ITDA, Parvathipuram, (unpublished).

Raj Pramukh, K.E. (2005), "The Shaman in Asia Pacific Region, A Cross-cultural study," *Man in India*, 85 (1&2), 25-40.

Rappaport, R.N. (1963), Discussion of S. Polgars Paper on Health of Human Behaviour. Curr. Anthro., 3, No. 2, 159-205.

Read, M. (1966), "Culture, Health aud Disease: Social and Cultural Influences on Health Programmes in Developing Countries", London: Tavistock.

Riesenfeld, A. (1950), The Megalithic Culture of Melanesia, Lieden.

Rojel (1953), The Interrelation between Uterine Cancer and Syphilis, Acta. Pathol. Microbial-Scand. Supp., 97:3.

Roth, H. Ling (1896), The Natives of Sarawak and British North Borneo, Mss. London.

Randy , R.W. (1978), "A Model for Combining Human Behaviour and Diseases Ecology to Assess Disease Hazards in a Community: Rural Ethiopia as a Model", Soc. Sci . Med., Ann Amer. Acad. P.A Soc. Sci., 346:334.

Rubel (1964), The Epidemiology of a Folk Illness: Susto in Hisponic America, Ethnology 3:268-83.

Sandisan, A.T. (1980), "Diseases in Ancient Egypt" in Mummies, Disease and Ancient Cultures (ed.) Aiden and Eve Cockburn, Cambridge University Press, Cambridge.

Schafer, J. (1989), "Utilizing Indigenous Agricultural Knowledge in the Planning of Agricultural Research Projects Designed to Aid Small Scale Farmers," in Indigenous Knowledge Systems: Implications for Agriculture and International Development Ed. by D. M. Warren, L.J. Slikkerveer, and S.O. Tittlola. Ames: Iowa State University.

Scotch, N. and H.J. Geiger (1962), The Epidemiology of Rheumatoid Arthritis: A Review with Special Attention to Social Factors, J. Chron, dis., 15:1037-1067.

Scotch, A. Norman (1963), Medicial Anthropology. Biennial Review of Anthropology, Stanford University Press, Stanford, California, pp. 39-40.

Geiger, H.J. and N.A. Scotch (1963), The Epidemiology of Essential Hypertension: A Receive with Special Attention to Psychological and Socio-cultural Factors, I. Biological Mechanism and Descriptive Epidemiology, II. Psychologic and Socio-cultural Factors in Etiology, *J. Chron dis.*

Selignan C.G. (1910), The Melanesians of British New Guinea, Cambridge.

Shiloh (1965), A Case Study of Desease and Culture in Action: Leprosy among the Hausa of Northern Nigeria, Hum. Organization 24: 140-47.

Sillitoe, Paul (1998), "The Development of Indigenous Knowledge", *Current Anthropology,* 39: 223-53.

Skeat, W.W. (1900), Malay Magic, London.

Smith, Bryan (1979), Community Health: An Epidemiological Approach, Mc. Millan, New York.

Suess, M.J. (1982), Examination of Water for Pollution Control (1&2), WHO Pergaman Press.

Tambiah, Stanley (1990), Magic, Science, and the Scope of Rationality, Cambridge: University Press.

Tataryn, J. (2002), Paradigms of Health and Disease. A Framework for Classifying and Understanding Complementary and Alternative Medicine, *Journal of Altern Complementary Medicine,* Dec. 8(6):893-95.

Turner, D.F. (1959), "Handbook of Diet Therapy", University of Chicago Press.

Tylor (1871), Primitive Culture.

Tenzel (1970), Shamanism and concepts of disease in a Malayan Indian Community, Psychiatry 33:372-80.

Von Mering and Kasdan (1970), Anthropology and the Behavioural and Health Sciences, University of Pittsburg Press, Pittsburg.

UNAIDS, (2006), *Report on the Global AIDS Epidemic.*

Vogel, V.J. (1970), "American Indian Medicine", Norman: University of Oklahama Press.

Varela, Thomsan, Rosely E. (1991), The Embodied Mind: Cognitive Science, Cambridge, HIT Press.

Weiss, M.G. (1985), The Interrelationship of Tropical Disease and Mental Disorder: Conceptual Framework and Literature Review, Part-I, Malaria, Culture, Med. Psychiatry, 9, 121-200.

WHO (1971), International Standards for Drinking Water, (3rd Ed.) World Health Organization, Geneva.

Wilson, P.J. (1967), Status Ambiguity and Spirit Possession, Man, 2, 366-78.

Wootton, David (2006), Bad Medicine: Doctors doing harm since Hippocrates, Oxford.

Young, Allan (1982), The Anthropologies of Illness and Sickness. Ann. Rev. Anthrop, 11:257–285.

INDEX